To our teachers.

Through word and example,

they have shown us

that when we cherish one another's gifts,

the world becomes a better, brighter place

Acknowledgments

This project has come about through the efforts of many people. Those who laid the philosophical groundwork for the One Candle Power process are mentioned within the text itself. Some I know personally; others I know only by reputation. Either way, they have changed countless lives through their vision of community and interdependence, and I owe them an enormous debt of gratitude.

Pat Beeman, George Ducharme, and Beth Mount brought these ideas to Connecticut and made them a reality for people here. They not only developed the monographs which gave rise to this volume, but lived these principles every day as a way to make the world a better place for everyone.

Putting this book together would not have been possible without much support and cooperation. Pat and George held my hand as I planned and worried and wrote and worried some more. Debbie Barisano and Camilla Dudley made phone calls, transcribed interviews from cassette, did proofreading and typing, and turned a lot of pages for me. A number of people shared their stories, either by writing them down or by agreeing to be interviewed. The people at Co-op Initiatives allowed me to put other projects aside and focus only on the development of this document. Therese Nadeau and Betsy Crum have been strong in their support for me. Thanks to all for the part you played in this process.

Since it is impossible to read one's own work objectively, I asked a number of people to respond to a draft. Some of them invited others as well. These diligent souls were Debbie Barisano, Jane Barrera, Pat Beeman, Curt Curtin, Regina DeMarasse, George Ducharme, Camilla Dudley,

ONE CANDLE POWER

Seven Principles
That Enhance the Lives
of People with Disabilities
and Their Communities

Based on the
One Candle Power
series from
Communitas

Revised by Cathy Ludlum,
with illustrations from her life
and the lives of others

Published by:

Inclusion Press International

24 Thome Crescent
Toronto,• Ontario • M6H 2S5 • CANADA
Phone: 416-658-5363 • Fax: 416-658-5067
WEB: www.inclusion.com
E-mail: info@inclusion.com

with

Communitas, Inc.

P. O. Box 358
Manchester, CT 06045-0358 USA
860-645-6976

National Library of Canada Cataloguing in Publication

One candle power: seven principles that enhance the lives of people with disabilities and their communities: based on the One candle power series by Communitas, /revised by Cathy Ludlum with illustrations from her life and the lives of others.

Based on 7 monographs published between 1988 and 1993 by Communitas.
ISBN 1-895418-48-8

1. People with disabilities--Services for.
I. Ludlum, Cathy
II. Communitas Inc.

HV1568.054 2002   362.4'048   C2002-904993-8

Janice Friedman, Eileen Furey, Bob Gorman, Mary Hough-Scholl, Cate Ludlam, Beth MacArthur, Linda Mead, Linda Meadows, Beth Mount, Dee O'Connor, Fr. Bill Olesik, Ernie Pancsofar, Timmy Randazzo, Julie Townsend, Katie Wolf, Lorie Zackin, Phyllis Zlotnick, . Their discovery of my typos and deep thoughts about larger issues improved this book greatly, and I appreciate the time and care they put in during the hectic summer season.

In addition, I thank all the people who helped to sponsor the publication of this book (see detailed list on the next page). My appreciation also goes to Jay Klein, whose support for this effort began many years ago. Natasha Bogdanova began work on the layout, and Jack Pearpoint completed it. Thanks to Communitas, Inc. and Inclusion Press International for publishing this volume.

Last, but by no means least, I want to thank the members of my circle of support for the many things they have made possible in my life over the years, including the development of this book. Their commitment to pursue my dreams along with me, combined with their constant encouragement and practical assistance, has allowed me to escape institutionalization and do some amazing things. This book attempts to describe that process in the hope that others will benefit from what we have learned.

Thanks to one and all!

Sponsors
Publication of this book was made possible in part by donations from…

Ms. Ethel Austin
Ms. Joyce Baker
Ms. Debbie Barisano
Ms. Patricia Beeman
Ms. Arlene Blum
Michael and Suzanne Bocchini
Ms. Leslie Burkhart
Rev. John and Maggie Carr
Karen and Eric Christensen
Dr. Bernie and Andrea Clark
Ms. Susan Coscia
Betsy Crum and Matt Guarino
Ms. Regina DeMarasse
George Ducharme, Ph.D.
Camilla and Earl Dudley
Rhonda and Lawrence Dvorin
Mr. Paul Ford
Mr. and Mrs. Daniel Friedman
Eileen Furey, Ph.D and Shirley Boron
Ms. Kathleen Gorman
Ms. Joanne Gray
Mr. David Guttchen
Rosemarie and Irv Hargrave
Mr. David Hogan
Ms. Michele Jordan
Ms. Marijke Kehrhahn
Susan and Richard King
Stan and Carol Kosloski
Cathleen Kowalski, D.M.D.
Claire and John Langton
Deborah and Larry Levine
Ms. Diane Libbey
Mrs. Shirley Lindberg
The Lozano Family

Charles Ludlum and Jane Gaylord
Dr. David and Carlene Ludlum
Ms. Meg Ludlum
William and Barbara Ludlum
Ms. Diane Mansfield
Gary and Kathy McDonough
Ms. Jane McNichol
Ms. Linda Mead
The Meadows Family
Phyllis and Arnold Mendelsohn
Judy and Harold Meyer
Ms. Joy Minervini
Ms. Lucille Morrissette
Mr. Peter Morrissette
Ms. Rosalie Newman
Dee O'Connor and Curt Curtin
Ms. Judith Ortiz
Ms. Amy Porter
Beverly and Edward Posusney
Mr. Ed Preneta
Mrs. Timmy Randazzo
Ms. Jane Reardon
Dr. Paul Scalise
Michael and Barbara Snyder
Mr. and Mrs. Allen Thompson
Representative John Thompson and Mrs. Elizabeth Thompson
Julie Townsend and Peter Love
Russell and Jean Tupper
Mr. Michael Valuckas
Ms. Roselle Weiner
Ms. Sharon Woodley
Jean and Roy Wrenn
Mr. and Mrs. Walter Zawacki
Ms. Phyllis Zlotnick

Thank You.   Your generosity makes this and future projects possible.

"It is better to light one candle

than to curse the darkness."

-- The Christophers

One Candle Power

You may not have heard the term, but it is likely that you have had the experience. You might have been at Girl Scout or Boy Scout Camp, at Midnight Mass, or at a vigil for a cause or in memory of someone...

As you arrive, you are given a candle. You stand in the darkness with your fellow scouts, or congregants, or neighbors, holding the cold stick of wax. Words are spoken: words of welcome or of farewell... words of comfort and healing... words of hope...

Then someone lights the first candle, gazes at the tiny flame for a moment, then touches it to the wick being held by the next person. That person lights the candle of another, who kindles another. The flame comes your way, and the person beside you reaches over to light your candle. You turn and share the light with the person on your other side. And so it goes. There may be the silence of shared awe, or there may be a song...

The room or clearing, which had seemed so dark before, has become a warmer and friendlier place as the faces glow in the flickering candlelight. Each person is separate; yet all are united.

A sudden gust of wind may disrupt the moment by blowing out a few of the candles. Disappointment, loneliness, sorrow, and exhaustion sometimes blow into our lives in a similar way. But not to worry; others are nearby to rekindle the light and to offer a smile of encouragement.

There is something profound in this simple ritual. As ancient as fire, yet as new as the youngest person in the group, it symbolizes a number of truths. It represents community at its best. It demonstrates that every person belongs and is significant. And it shows that when you share your flame – your gift – with another person, it is in no way diminished. Instead, it is multiplied.

Throughout this book, we will be using the expression One Candle Power to capture the idea that every person brings a unique gift to the world. This is as true of people with disabilities as it is of other members of society. This gift needs to be shared with our fellow human beings. By a willingness to offer our own gift and to seek and accept the gifts of others, each of us becomes a fuller person, richer in experience and more vibrantly alive.

Table of Contents

PART I: THE SEVEN STRATEGIES

BUILDING BRIDGES

STARTING SMALL

CHANGING SYSTEMS

PART II: IMPERFECT CHANGE

DON'T FORGET TO HAVE FUN

RESOURCES

INTRODUCTION

In the fall of 1986, I attended a conference sponsored by Northspring Consulting (which later became Communitas, Inc.) with funding from the Connecticut Council on Developmental Disabilities. The conference organizers, George Ducharme, Ph.D., and Pat Beeman, had spent years researching ways people with disabilities could live in communities as valued and participating members. Until that time, people usually resided in institutions or with aging parents; or they lived an isolated existence in the community as recipients of services, but still not as full citizens.

Pat and George, as they came to be known, invited three speakers to their conference to describe innovative methods of community inclusion.

- John McKnight, of Northwestern University in Chicago, startled us with the idea that paid supports, while important, are not really the key to independence. Whether we have disabilities or not, what makes us safe, successful, and happy is surrounding ourselves with people who care about us.
- David Wetherow, from the Prairie Housing Cooperative in Winnipeg, Canada, introduced us to people with severe disabilities who were living in environments of mutual support and full participation in different parts of his city.
- Beth Mount, Ph.D., from Graphic Futures in Atlanta, literally drew the lives of real people as a way to make their lives better. Vivid magic-marker pictures, filled with rainbows and circles of people, brought us deep into stories of difficulty and triumph. And Beth didn't just draw the past; her art helped to change the future!

While at the conference I saw a number of people I knew. Mary-Ann Langton and I had been friends since we were teenagers. She was there with her mom, Claire. Kevin

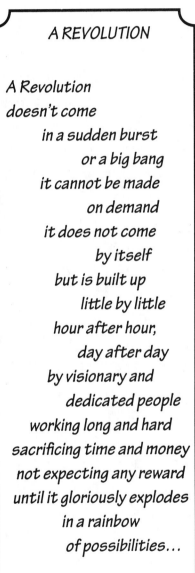

A REVOLUTION

A Revolution
doesn't come
in a sudden burst
or a big bang
it cannot be made
on demand
it does not come
by itself
but is built up
little by little
hour after hour,
day after day
by visionary and
dedicated people
working long and hard
sacrificing time and money
not expecting any reward
until it gloriously explodes
in a rainbow
of possibilities...

Angel Nieto Romero

Meadows and I went to school together as kids, but had fallen out-of-touch after I graduated. He and his mother, Linda, and I renewed our friendship in between conference sessions. Todd Kilroy was a fellow disability rights advocate. Each of us brought different perspectives and goals. Even so, it is no exaggeration to say that what happened over those three days changed our lives.

In January of 1987, five individuals and families were selected to begin trying out the principles described at the conference. One element, circles of support, became especially popular. A circle is a problem-solving process which involves family and friends to support a person in pursuing a vision of the future. A complete description appears in the Seven Strategies section of this book. By June of 1988 there were 25 circles working on housing, school, employment, and a variety of other issues. Each circle chose its own direction based on the wishes of the member with a disability.

Before long, we were invited to speak to small informal groups and to write about what we were learning. Pat and George, together with Beth Mount, believed that those of us with disabilities and our families should be considered the "experts" and be invited to speak on our own behalf. This was a revolutionary concept at a time when disability conferences were still being conducted by professionals, and without any people with disabilities present.

Then George became President-elect of the Northeast Region of what was then called the American Association on Mental Deficiency (now the American Association on Mental Retardation). As a result, he and Pat coordinated a full-scale conference, and included speakers with disabilities in every conference session and keynote presentation. It was a controversial move at the time, but eventually it caught on in other places.

So off we went to other conferences – in twos and threes, and sometimes in a larger contingent – to tell how we were becoming involved in our communities and, through that process, finding the support we needed. It seemed that people everywhere were hungry for this message.

The following year Pat, Beth, and George began to write a series of monographs which outlined the concepts of community inclusion, circles of support, recognizing each person's gifts, and building bridges to community life. They continued their tradition of empowerment by encouraging us to submit our own stories and observations. Eventually, seven monographs were developed; they became known collectively as the *One Candle Power* series:

- *One Candle Power: Building Bridges into Community Life for People with Disabilities*
- *What Are We Learning about Bridge-Building?*
- *What Are We Learning about Circles of Support?*
- *Person-Centered Development: A Journey in Learning to Listen to People with Disabilities*
- *Dare to Dream: An Analysis of the Conditions Leading to Personal Change for People with Disabilities*
- *Imperfect Change: Embracing the Tensions of Person-Centered Work*
- *Tending the Candle: A Booklet for Circle Facilitators*

For several years now, Pat and George have been talking about updating this series. We have all learned so much since the monographs were written in the late 1980s and early 1990s. The basic principles still hold true, and we have seen them at work over time, through victory, through tragedy, and even through death.

Revising the series has long been a dream of mine, and now the timing seems right. In this volume, we will revisit the One Candle Power concept. Through its seven components, the lives of people with disabilities as well as the lives of our communities have been enriched. As always, stories are used to bring these principles to life.

People often talk about me as an example of success in using these methods to gain independence, connection, and happiness in my life, so my story is included throughout to illustrate many of the points. Many people who do not know me well do not realize how close I came to entering a nursing home. They are not aware of how many times having an organized network of close and proactive friends has literally saved my life. If I have been able to give my gift to the world, it is because I have been well-supported in living independently (and in simply living at all). These circumstances are part of the story, too.

Sir Isaac Newton said, "If I have seen further, it is by standing on the shoulders of giants." I have had the privilege of seeing how one candle -- one idea or relationship or experience -- can bring light to others, even as it lights the way of the solitary traveler. I have seen people come together in times of joy and in times of distress to support one another as they press on toward the dream. It has been a privilege to be part of something so important and so wonderful.

Throughout this book, you will notice statements like "We have learned…." or "It has been our experience…." Who are "we"? Since I am building on the work of Pat, Beth, and George, part of the answer is the four of us. But it is not limited to us. Having listened to many other people involved with circles of support, bridge-building, and the other One Candle Power strategies, I am trying to relate a communal outlook we have all acquired through our shared experiences.

We offer the following information, not as authorities, but as people in the process of learning together. We are standing, with you, on the shoulders of giants as we all blaze the way for future generations…

Cathy Ludlum
Manchester, Connecticut
November 7, 2002

FOUNDERS AND FRAMEWORK

One Candle Power began as a process centered on a person with a disability, his or her vision of the future, and family, friends, and interested professionals who gathered to walk along with the person as fellow travelers. Over the years, the wisdom of this method has been understood by people without disabilities as well, so the process has achieved a more generic use. This represents the swing of the pendulum back from the desire for total independence (which can sometimes result in isolation) toward a model which supports independence through interdependence.

The candle was chosen as a symbol because of its simplicity, ease of use, ancient heritage, yet current practicality: when modern lighting technology fails, we return to the candle. Its endless symbolic interpretations help us illustrate the concepts of supporting, empowering, and "shining a light" on people and their sometimes-hidden gifts and abilities. This applies, not only to people with disabilities themselves, but to the members of their social networks and their communities as well.

The One Candle Power process was created through the gifts of many people whose teachings have inspired us. We began by:

- Adopting the principles of capacity-seeking and capacity-building articulated by David Wetherow, John McKnight, Beth Mount, John O'Brien and Robert Rodale;

- Using the Personal Futures Planning approach developed by Beth Mount;

- Building upon the experiences of Judith Snow, Peter Dill, Marsha Forest and Jack Pearpoint in creating the first circles of support in Toronto, Canada;

♦ Using and encouraging the use of the bridge-building techniques described by John McKnight and practiced by many people throughout the United States and Canada;

♦ Believing in the power of one candle as articulated by the Christophers: "It is better to light one candle than to curse the darkness;"

♦ Accepting the basic truth lived and described by Jean Vanier and the people of the L'Arche communities and the Faith and Light movement: that the gift of every person, no matter what label he or she may have, is unique and of great value;

♦ Believing that the people in local community associations will show hospitality and acceptance to people with disabilities who are introduced to them by friends, as articulated by John McKnight, Ivan Illich, Parker Palmer, Henri Nouwen, Alexis DeToqueville, and Robert Bellah; and

♦ Accepting the truth of the paradox that states: "If we give our flame or gift to another, our flame or gift will not be diminished; but in fact, the result will be the opposite. There will be more light!"

> *A single thread takes on new meaning when it is interwoven with other diverse threads. Distinct and vibrant on its own, it becomes an essential part of something much greater than itself.*
>
> *Unknown*

When the seven books in the *One Candle Power* series came out (from 1988 through 1993), we were just beginning to understand the effect individuals and their communities could have upon one another. Over the years, we have learned more, but the original material has not become out-of-date. Some volumes have sold out, yet individuals, family members, service providers, community folks, and college professors still contact Communitas in search of these books.

In "The Seven Strategies," Part I of this book, we are reproducing the first three monographs from the original *One Candle Power* series. This collection of road maps, assumptions, and stories has been used by many people over the last 14 years. Since much was written about circles of support, and this continues to be the most well-known element of the One Candle Power process, the section about circles is significantly longer than other parts of this book. Much of the original "how-to" information is still there. Material that was repeated among the various monographs has been removed, and new insights and stories have been added here and there. But it has been a happy surprise to discover that the documents, *as we produced them,* are still so relevant. If you have used the old series and become attached to it, you will find much that seems familiar in these pages.

The second section, "Imperfect Change," carries the title of one of the most popular monographs. Although the One Candle Power principles do work, nobody said this process was going to be easy. Relationships fracture. People die. Community can sometimes be ugly. Funding for community-based services is hard to come by; and even after you get it, sometimes the budget is cut and programs are eliminated. Saying this out loud and in writing has somehow been comforting to people.

Also in Part II, you will learn what became of many of the people you met through the first series. You will also get acquainted with some new people whose journeys give us additional perspective. These stories shed light on the deeper implications of community, interdependence, and autonomy. As the tables are turned, people with disabilities have become caregivers for elderly parents, and unfulfilled dreams of community have led to the creation of new informal networks.

Over the years, Communitas has produced, obtained, or heard about a number of documents and audio and video tapes that also expand on these concepts. An extensive bibliography of additional resources, people and organizations is included at the end of this book.

Every situation of personal and community change is different and demands a unique response. We have identified seven strategies that can be used consistently and combined in countless ways according to the situation. Our understanding of how to use these concepts has evolved since our journey of walking with people began in 1987. This document contains the best of what we know about supporting personal, community, organizational, and policy change for people with disabilities.

We encourage you to use these strategies and resources in ways that fit the unique challenges you face.

OVERVIEW:
THE ONE CANDLE POWER PROCESS

Traditionally, people with disabilities have been weighed down by the perceptions of others. They have been treated as collections of problems, rather than as people with strengths as well as weaknesses. Their choices have been limited, either because they have not been allowed to make their own decisions, or because few options have been offered. When people have dared to express their dreams, of going to a regular high school, getting a satisfying job, or having their own home, their dreams have been called "unrealistic." Often, people with disabilities have been pulled out of communities, into special schools, sheltered workshops, and residential institutions because this was thought to be the most effective way to meet their needs.

The One Candle Power process makes it possible for us to leave the darkness of these old assumptions, and to emerge into a world where there is more light and opportunity.

One Candle Power begins when one person has an idea so compelling that others are drawn in, and together they begin to create change. The idea may come from the person him- or herself through the frustration of hitting dead ends in pursuit of a goal. Or it may come from someone who has been **walking with** the person, and realizing that something could be better in his or her life. The objective may be modest, such as three people gathering to help someone participate in the local bridge club. Change may grow as people notice the success and want to light a candle in their own neighborhood.

The process centers around the person him- or herself, and this person is often referred to as the **focus person**. Although limitations are recognized, the emphasis is always on his or her **capacities**. Society typically views the

ONE CANDLE POWER IS ABOUT:

- HOPE
- DREAMS
- CAPACITIES
- TAKING RISKS
- BREAKING NEW GROUND
- WALKING WITH
- BUILDING RELATIONSHIPS
- PRESENCE AND RESPONSIVENESS
- INTERDEPENDENCE
- EMPOWERMENT
- LISTENING
- HELPING EACH OTHER TO GROW
- SLOWING DOWN TO BE WITH ONE ANOTHER
- ALLOWING TIME FOR THINGS TO HAPPEN

person with a disability as in need of help; but concentrating on capacities allows us to see what the person can offer to others. Gifts such as a sense of humor, a talent for listening, or an ability to bring people together cause friends and community members to seek him or her out, and the result is that everyone wins.

The focus person has the authority to decide what will work best. His or her **vision** is taken seriously, and everything in the One Candle Power process is connected somehow to the pursuit of that vision. One means of pursuing the vision is to create a **circle of support**. The circle consists of the people the focus person has chosen to bring along on his or her journey toward the vision. Typically, circle members come from family, school, workplace, religious affiliation, or neighborhood. Service providers may be included, but the emphasis is on people who have natural ties to or share common interests with the person. Although circle meetings are filled with energetic brainstorming, and while dozens of suggestions may be generated, the focus person chooses which ideas will be carried out and how the group process will proceed.

The local community has been an underutilized source of ideas and support. **Building bridges** to the community is key to ending isolation, increasing involvement, and ultimately reaching the dream. For example, someone who is interested in music may want to find out when and where concerts are held. With a town newspaper and phone book, circle members can gather preliminary information about events and resources, and then the focus person can determine what happens next. If transportation or support is needed, consider natural connections first, such as a circle member tagging along to get things started. This may lead to a carpooling arrangement with someone in the organization and the possibility of a new friendship.

In working toward the vision, it's okay to **start small**. Every little step does count, and minor victories ward off

> Conversation is the natural way humans think together.
>
> Margaret Wheatley,
> Turning to One Another

3

frustration and boredom as the friends wait for the wheels of bureaucracy to turn, the eligibility period to go by, or the new home to be ready.

Sometimes attaining a vision will require changing systems which already exist. Service systems and other large entities have sometimes been made more responsive by circle members who were committed to a vision and simply unwilling to give up.

Walking With

At a time when quick is beautiful, and fast food, automatic teller machines, and email have become a way of life, it is difficult to slow down enough to really be with people. Yet the best metaphor to describe the One Candle Power process is that of a journey: a journey which may be shared for a lifetime. We travel at a walking pace. The importance of this journey is not so much its destination (although that too has its place), but the interactions of people from day to day and from moment to moment.

The following article, written by George Ducharme and Pat Beeman, is adapted from the Spring 1991 issue of the **Communitas Communicator**.

Walking With

"Walking with" someone means
Accepting the person where he or she is at right now
Walking at the pace the person wants to walk
Working "in partnership with" rather than "doing for"
Not trying to fix or control the person

This is what we have experienced as we have had the pleasure of "walking with" a number of people with disabilities and their families.

Although every situation is different, certain themes stand out. The vision of the person may be difficult to reach. We often find ourselves going down untravelled paths that bring times of tension and struggle. But the important thing is to continue striving to come as close to the vision as possible. Obstacles may stand in the way, but opportunities also present themselves, and in between we just walk along together.

"Walking with" requires **commitment.**

"Commitment is what transforms
a promise into reality.
It is the words that speak boldly of your intentions.
And the actions which speak louder than the words.

"It is making the time when there is none.
Coming through time after time,
year after year after year.

"Commitment is the stuff character is made of,
the power to change the face of things.

"It is the daily triumph of integrity over skepticism."

(a poem given to us by a friend)

**"Walking with" requires
presence and responsiveness.**

The notion of simply "being there" as a human "being," not a human "doing" is a very important notion. But it is hard to understand and do. You can be present for someone when he or she is going through a rough spot, be there when no one else is, be there sometimes at your own life's expense, and it may not be to do anything but BE.

Time drags for those who wait for agencies, services, and people. Be present. Support them. Give a call, write a note, stop by, and help troubleshoot. Caring means being present to each other.

We have discovered that "walking with" someone is not a very complicated or a very new idea. Being committed, being present, and being responsive are all simple, age-old activities. In today's society, however, we are constantly encouraged to ride the fast track and to look out for Number One. Take the opportunity to swim against the tide!

WE RECOMMEND A GOOD WALK WITH ANOTHER.

IT'LL BE GOOD FOR BOTH OF YOU!

It's not differences that divide us. It's our judgments about each other that do.

*Margaret Wheatley,
Turning to One Another*

LEADERSHIP

The Power of One

Sometimes don't you feel like you're out there all alone
Working hard on so much to get done.
You're tired and discouraged
And you just don't have the time to notice you're the power of one.

Chorus
It's the power of one,
To do what you can do
To dream a better future and to know
That whenever someone starts to do what they can do
Then the power of one can grow

Oh, maybe you are someone who's looking for a friend
For yourself, for your daughter, or your son.
You've dreamed and you've struggled,
And now it's time to know
That you really are the power of one.

Chorus

It's a little like you're going
Through a field of underbrush
Hacking out a path for more to come,
Or maybe you're a candle that lights the darkened room
With light that's from the power of one.

Chorus

When somebody says you can't do things that way
'Cause after all you're only one
Remind them that changes mostly happen step by step
And often from the power of one.

Chorus

So the power of one becomes two or three
And two or three become ninety one,
And then you look around to see how things have changed
Just because you were the power of one.

Chorus

Yes, the power of one can grow!

© 1991 Tom Hunter
With thanks to Patty Gerdel and the Beach Center
Full Citizenship Great Expectations Summer Institute

IT ALL BEGINS
WITH A *GOOD* LEADER

The most famous aspect of the One Candle Power process is the circle of support. Members of a circle come together to enhance the life of someone they care about, often a person with a disability or a family in which one or more of the members has a disability. You will read more about circles beginning on page 46.

But a circle does not just happen, and neither do the other aspects of One Candle Power (such as creating a vision of the future or changing a service system). Even though many people are needed to effect the change, someone needs to initiate the process, provide followup, and coordinate the activities over time.

The leader may have a disability, and be seeking to create a better future for him- or herself. Or the leader may bring several people together in a spirit of concern and collaboration with a family member with a disability. However it starts, the process of bringing about lasting change involves some or all of the following methods:

♦ **Finding a Vision and Planning a Future**

♦ **Building on Capacities**

♦ **Building Circles of Support**

♦ **Building Bridges to Community Life**

♦ **Starting Small**

♦ **Changing Systems**

Some people are natural leaders. Others may shrink back, feeling inadequate to take on this role. But many

> If you have come to help me you are wasting your time, but if you have come because your liberation is bound up with mine, then let us speak together.
>
> - Lila Watson

people have the ability hidden within them, and concern for someone's well-being may bring it out.

The ability of a group to move forward through the process of One Candle Power depends on having an effective leader. Here are some thoughts about leadership that are useful in bringing about change.

Qualities of Effective Leaders

Effective leaders have vastly different personalities, approaches, and techniques, but we find that they share certain values and qualities.

Effective leaders:

♦ **SEE CAPACITIES** in every person; recognize all people as gifted

♦ **TRUST IN PEOPLE'S CAPACITY TO KNOW** what they want, and how to make that happen in a positive way

♦ **INSPIRE COOPERATION AND ACTION**

♦ **USE CREATIVITY** to suggest new directions and new combinations of ideas

♦ **SEE SMALL AND SIMPLE AS BEAUTIFUL**

An effective leader is crucial to the success of a circle of support. Circles work best when all the members of the circle feel empowered to take actions that will benefit the focus person. The ability of a group to identify how to proceed, to find creative avenues for change, and to cooperate in making things happen depends on good leadership.

A circle leader can be an unpaid, committed ally, such as a friend, family member, or the person with a disability him/herself. Or the leader may be a paid facilitator, professional, or other interested person.

Effective leaders do not pre-judge another person's gift (their candle power). Those who might be dismissed as having "little to give" may well surprise us if we continue to support and nurture the light within them.

Effective Leaders See Capacities

An effective leader sees an individual with a label as a gifted person, regardless of any real or perceived limitations. Not only does the leader recognize the gifts within the focus person; the leader can also see how much the larger community could benefit if these gifts were liberated and channeled into community life. In addition, an effective leader is aware of the gifts of each member in a circle of support, and finds ways for each person to contribute in the process of change.

Individual gifts within a group may be given in many different ways. Some members contribute ideas during circle meetings. Others offer emotional support over the phone and in day-to-day problem solving. Some people like to take concrete action while others provide inspiration and encouragement. A good leader recognizes these preferences and supports each type of individual contribution.

> As for the best leaders, the people do not notice their existence…
> When the best leader's work is done, the people say, "We did it ourselves!"
> - Lao-tzu

Effective Leaders Trust in People's Capacity to Know

Effective leaders believe that there is a deep and abiding wisdom in all people, and they know how to harness this wisdom to benefit the person with a disability. An effective leader understands that people with degrees and professional standing are not the only people with knowledge. They realize that people with disabilities, their moms and dads, brothers and sisters, neighbors, co-workers, and fellow members of clubs or religious organizations often have real wisdom about the life of the community and how to make things happen.

The skills and talents of ordinary folks provide a reservoir of energy and power needed to build a better life for community members who need extra support. A good leader knows that power is there, and understands how to stimulate the extraordinary wisdom and action of ordinary people.

Effective Leaders Inspire Cooperation and Action

An effective leader inspires cooperation among network members in working together to build new possibilities. The lessons taught by those who use non-competitive, cooperative approaches are important to the One Candle Power process. Clearly, this is not a place for competitive struggles. Circles of support allow individuals to give their best gifts to one another. It is centered, therefore, not on competition but on enhancing the gifts of others.

The words and struggles of Martin Luther King, Jr., Gandhi, Lech Walesa, Mother Teresa, Jean Vanier and others form the philosophical base for this structure. Individuals may be assertive and persistent in pursuit of dreams and the elimination of injustice, but winning is not the objective here. Everyone has the ability to give his or her gift and help to move the process forward. A good leader supports people in doing that.

Effective Leaders Use Creativity

One of the greatest deterrents to reaching a person's dream is a locked mind. Being able to create new combinations or to explore new paths is an important part of this process. An effective leader has the ability to help people explore new possibilities from the information, resources, and opportunities suggested by each person. For most of the people we have met over the last 15 years, the

> *The reasonable man adapts himself to the world, the unreasonable one persists in trying to adapt the world to himself. Therefore, all progress depends upon the unreasonable man.*
>
> *- George Bernard Shaw*

best gift we could give was to offer new ways of thinking about and working on their dream.

Effective Leaders See Small and Simple As Beautiful

An effective leader knows how to start small and to value every simple act that moves the process forward. In the pursuit of big dreams and in the face of complex realities, it is important to proceed a little at a time to avoid becoming overwhelmed and discouraged.

The good leader attempts to make the process of change as simple as possible. Participation is needed from both the most educated person as well as the person who speaks directly from the heart. The leader recognizes the inherent dignity and capacity of each person, and promotes a process that enables everyone to participate. The leader builds on existing resources within communities and within people without waiting for something outside to "save the day."

> We can do no great things; only small things with great love.
>
> - Mother Teresa

In the final analysis, true leadership lies in the ability to focus the gifts of others so that all may benefit. The next story illustrates how leadership is often taught by example. The second story emphasizes that leaders need to be watching for the capacities in people, even when those capacities may not be apparent at first.

GROWING UP AROUND ADVOCACY

Mary-Ann Langton

As a child, I learned what advocacy was by watching my mom. Mom was (and is) a strong advocate for me, but also for all people with disabilities. In junior high school I began to realize that if I was going to wait for other people to advocate for me, I would not get anywhere in life.

Mom first taught me the importance of advocacy through my IEP (Individualized Education Plan) process. She became tired of going to meetings and getting information from the teachers, then coming home and telling me everything that had gone on. I would listen to her description of what they said about me, and I would say, "Mom, it's not true." The first time I went to my IEP meeting with my mom, she did not tell them I would be coming. The eyes on my teachers grew wide because they were shocked that a student with a disability as severe as mine could speak and disagree with them. It took a couple of years for the teachers to learn I could (and would) disagree with their recommendations. My mom and I were a great team because we were able to play off of one another.

Then Mom was invited to be on the Connecticut Council on Developmental Disabilities, a Governor-appointed council of individuals with disabilities, parents, and designated professionals who create policy change. Because I was in school, and the Council wanted to focus on inclusive education, my mom was honored and excited to be asked to join. Mom did not make all the Council meetings because I was either sick or, if my brother and sister were not available, she had to be home to get me off the school bus. Since Mom had difficulty attending the Council meetings, she found other ways to participate. She was always on the phone catching up on what happened and giving her input. After awhile, my mom became very involved in a committee; the way she could be so involved was that the committee met in our dining room. So mom could run out and get me off the bus, bring me in, set me up, and then return to the dining room and participate in the committee. That went on for years, and I got to know the Council members. They were always so nice when I came in from school, saying "Hi, how are you?" All I could think was, "Just let me go into my room and hide!" But little by little I got to know them, and when I got older I was invited to be on the Council myself.

So my mom and I were both council members at the same time, but everyone treated us as individuals. It didn't take people long to see that we had different ideas and different ways. I remember one time we had an overnight Council retreat, and my mom got sick right before we were supposed to go. Mom and I were always roommates at things like this. I called Maggie at the Council office, and said, "Oh my! I don't know what to do!" Maggie said she would make a few calls, and in the end another Council member said she would be my roommate and support me with anything I needed. She and I had more fun... we were up until late hours talking about her family and my family and everything else. I still keep in touch with her.

But still it was difficult for me to advocate for myself. I went to Council meetings and served on the Education Committee because that was my pet peeve. I remember meetings where I wanted to disagree with a committee member, but at first I was afraid to jump in. The chair always read my eyes. He would stop the conversation and say, "Mary-Ann wants to talk." I did not know who he was except that I knew his name. It turned out that he was the Deputy Commissioner of the Department of Mental Retardation.

Later, they asked me to be in charge of the committee! I was thinking, "Yeah, sure. Why me?" But I agreed to do it, and that meant I also had to attend executive committee meetings and my mom was not there. So I wondered, "Who will support me? Who will pick me up from college?" At this time, I was living in New Haven while I attended Southern Connecticut State University. Before I could get too concerned, one of the Council members who lived in the area said he would provide my transportation, and another member said she would help me with eating. It was all very natural. It was like a true community because we cared about one another. So it seems that along my walk there have been people nudging me forward so that I might become the person I am today.

After I graduated from college, I held many jobs in human services where I worked one-on-one with people with disabilities and sometimes with their parents. I was very excited when I went for my first job interview. I thought it would be a job I would love. When my boss met me, however, he freaked out. He could not deal with my disability. He could not (or would not) understand my speech. On my first day of work, he put my desk up against the wall so no one would see me. He gave me no work to do. Talk about boredom… I left that job before I got fired because I did not take much grief from people at that point.

I went to a job which involved welcoming all people with disabilities into faith communities. I loved this job. This was where I learned how important it was to collaborate with other people.

After this, I took another job where I worked with individuals with disabilities. Here again, however, I felt like my colleagues didn't see me. Instead, they saw my wheelchair and they saw what I could not do. I tried to ignore these attitudes and just focused on my work because I enjoyed the people that I was there to support. Through their lives and struggles, I saw the changes that needed to be made in transportation, PCA (personal care attendant) supports, housing, and advocacy in order for things to improve. It was here that I became more aware of the need to work on a systems level. I tried to get my Masters in Social Work, but that did not work out because of discrimination.

But at that time there was a job posted for a Disability Policy Specialist at the Council on Developmental Disabilities. Ed Preneta, who had been at the Council serving as Director since 1978, wanted to try something new because Maggie Carr was retiring. So Ed and the Council decided to divide up her salary and hire two people. One would be a person with a severe disability, and another would be a parent of a child with a developmental disability. When I saw the job I thought "This is a job I would love, but the state would not hire me." But I kept getting more copies of this job posting, and I finally decided "Why not try it?" It was like a dream. Because typing is difficult for me and there was a time limit for getting my resume in, I needed to rely on my circle of support. I called one of my friends and said "Would you type up a cover letter for me? I will tell you what I would like to say." So my friend came over and we had a lot of fun writing my cover letter. We mailed the letter together that day. Later, I got a call from Ed to set the time for my interview. My interview was wonderful! As Ed talked about what my job responsibilities would be, I was thinking,

"These are my gifts that I would like to share." I waited a couple of days while Ed checked on my references. On Saturday afternoon he called and offered me the job. I was shocked. Suddenly, I needed time to think about it because it would be such a change from working one-on-one to systems change. My family and my circle were very involved in my decisionmaking process. They saw many possibilities. Together we turned the barriers (like transportation) into practical solutions (like using a combination of mass transit and a driver I would hire).

So I accepted the job and I began in June of 2000. Besides working on systems change directly, I have been able to organize conferences about transportation and quality assurance as will as little focus groups working on systems issues. The Council does not see obstacles. We often see barriers, but barriers can turn into possibilities if we brainstorm. The Council office is housed in the same building as the Department of Mental Retardation, and I work on a wonderful floor where I'm able to meet many people. I've gotten to know some of the other people in our building, and have invited them over to my house. At work, I feel comfortable asking them to open my lunch or provide me with any little support I may need. This is a nice supplement to my long-term, paid support. I have hired someone to support me with paperwork such as filing, and to drive me to meetings. I have traveled to Texas with a friend for our annual conference. I think it has been a great awareness to DMR, to the whole community, and to the Council on Developmental Disabilities itself, to know that with the proper support, I am able to hold down a job.

I have reached this point because of the many, many people I have met through my life. These people have become my mentors because they have shown me their gifts. Some of them have disabilities also, but not all. It all works together for all of us. I have learned that I can do anything, but I need to have the support, and that support needs to be under my control. An important systems issue is that support money must follow each person, so that he or she can choose what is needed and how to be a contributor in this world. My parents, my family, and my many friends have supported me through all these years, and never saw my disability as the most important thing. That is why I could get to the place I am today.

LEARNING FROM ANGELO AND SARAH
Pat Beeman

For many years, I have been on a journey of building communities where truth and justice prevail, where all the strangers in our midst are accepted and welcomed, and where interdependence abounds. Caring and compassion with one another form the heart of this community. There are a number of travelers that I have met on this path who have helped me define what "building community" is all about. I have lived this journey through the hearts of these travelers. They have given me some valuable tools to carry with me, and have filled me with hope that things are possible if we support one another in the struggles and joys we encounter daily…

Angelo, a 26-year-old handsome young man, greeted me with a great smile and wave. Sarah, with her beautiful brown eyes and long brown hair, made gurgling sounds. She came toward me pulling at my clothes, hugging me, listening to Sesame Street music.

"How can I ever communicate with these two young adults?" I wondered. What was I supposed to be learning from them to get me to the next step in this process? How could I learn from people who don't communicate like I do, who at best grab me, and who knows what else they might do? But our meeting was not by chance. I had a lot to learn yet about how to really "listen" to people.

Angelo had a tendency to become violent if he was not able to get his point across. Sarah seemed to wander aimlessly, never focusing in directly on me, but hugging and grabbing at me and making noises, and throwing things. Although I didn't understand at first, they were inviting me to open my mind to other ways of communicating than just MY way. Still I wondered, "How will we ever have a meeting of the minds?" THAT'S IT: we won't. But we will have a meeting of the hearts if we can stay open to one another long enough. Here was my opportunity to learn how to become a good listener and a good observer, and how to meet people where they are at.

This is a journey of seeing beyond the surface. It is a journey in listening to the body and learning to communicate in ways other than what we are used to.

With Angelo there were many false starts. My lack of any knowledge of sign language combined with not knowing what provoked Angelo caused us to miscommunicate, especially in the beginning. Angelo's inability to express to me (and somewhat to himself) what he was feeling and the embarrassment this caused him resulted in his punching out walls, or running out of a restaurant and walking home. So for me it was a matter of perseverance – of not giving up – of always coming back – no matter what – to try to meet Angelo at his level. It was finding a way to communicate to Angelo "I care. I value you for who you are. I want to be a friend. I want to learn how to be in a relationship with you."

After six months, Angelo and I were finally just beginning to figure some things out between us. There was the time we were planning to go out to eat, and I didn't understand where he wanted to go. He jumped out of my moving car and walked home. The next week I returned, and he communicated to me that if I got a piece of paper he would draw me a map so I would know where I was going.

Angelo taught me a lot about forgiveness. He never held a grudge. Every time I came back he would smile, greet me, and say through his body language, "Let's try again."

This journey is not about understanding why people do what they do, but accepting them where they are, growing with it, and knowing one day both of your lives will be enriched by that meeting.

When I first met Sarah, there was no obvious means of communication. How could I relate to a 16-year-old woman whose body, movements, and behavior appeared to be more like those of a 2-year-old? Yet she also invited me to listen and find ways to communicate with her.

Soon after, facilitated communication came into Sarah's life, and she has been able to express to us many things about how her body works. Her most insightful statement was "My body doesn't listen to me and neither do you." So from that day forward our relationship has grown in many ways. Sarah went on to become an honor student in the local high school, and created disability awareness days at her school to educate and involve her peers.

This journey requires that we never settle for what seems obvious. There is much within each person, and we need to keep our minds and hearts open to receive what they are trying to communicate. This journey has taught me that this "building community" is about building a broader community than just our immediate selves. It is a journey about patience: about slowing down, taking the time to listen to people, and being with people. People have invaluable things to say, but you need to take the time to let them say it at their own pace.

FINDING CAPACITIES

It has been said that "Nobody is so poor that he or she has nothing to give, and nobody is so rich that he or she has nothing to receive." Real human dignity is found both in giving and in receiving, and there is a continuous mutuality between the two. This is true not only for individuals but for nations, cultures, and religious communities as well. Let's never give anything without asking ourselves what we are receiving from those to whom we give, and let's never receive anything without asking what we have to give to those from whom we receive.

No human being is perfect physically, emotionally, intellectually, or spiritually; but every person brings important gifts to community life. Understanding this has practical implications in how we view the people around us, and ultimately in how we treat them. Is the glass half empty? Or is it half full? As capacity-seekers, our job is to uncover and clarify people's gifts. When this process is successful, people have increasing opportunities to make their capacities more apparent. It is a process which builds on itself and has the potential to become a self-fulfilling prophecy.

The positive qualities of people with disabilities have traditionally been denied or ignored. For decades, many human services were focused on the negative characteristics that someone might display. John McKnight showed us that the field of human services often depended on the deficits in people to justify the delivery of programs. These programs might – or might not – actually help people. The paperwork that many human service workers completed to qualify for funding required workers to focus on what was wrong instead of looking at what was right. The result was that the gifts and capacities people might bring to community life were often completely overlooked.

Over the last few years, human service agencies have attempted to incorporate a more positive approach to

> There are two ways
> to live your life.
>
> One is as though
> nothing is a miracle.
>
> The other is as though
> everything is a miracle.
>
> - Albert Einstein

their processes of evaluation and service delivery. It is no longer shocking to have a case worker say, "Let's look at what is going right for you" as well as identifying problem areas. Funders, both private and public, are becoming more interested in building on people's capacities. There is a small but distinct push toward supporting people instead of trying to manage or fix them.

The old way of thinking is not gone, however. It remains in procedural guidelines that range from overprotective to domineering. It remains in people's tendency to think that the best way to have their needs (or the needs of their loved one) met is in the security of an institution. It remains in the need for states to request Medicaid waivers from the federal government to pay for services in the community, while institutional care is guaranteed without special paperwork. And it remains in the attitudes of some human service workers who cannot conceive of people with disabilities as equal and contributing citizens.

Furthermore, many members of the community still hold unconscious stereotypes which limit their ability to see capacity in people. When community members perceive people with disabilities through these stereotypes, they may treat adults as if they are children, assume they are incompetent, or flee because they consider them a menace. These assumptions, while not as prevalent as they once were, still close many doors to people with disabilities.

As capacity finders, therefore, we must become ruthless at locating and uncovering people's unique gifts, and presenting them in the most positive light possible. In other words, we must push back against service practices and community attitudes to help others see how competent people with disabilities can be when they have the opportunity to show off their capacities.

The next three stories demonstrate the power of perceptions – positive and negative – in shaping the lives of people, especially people with disabilities.

COIN STORY

Cathy Ludlum

I remember sitting on the floor of our apartment in New York City, surrounded by coins and paper coin rollers. We moved to Connecticut when I was five, so I must have been younger than that; and my sense is that I was quite a bit younger, perhaps even toward the end of my third year. My task was to take the coins and fit them into the coin rollers. At first I needed some help folding the paper ends in, and I am not sure when I took on the responsibility for actually counting the coins. With practice, however, I got to be good at this household chore.

Whenever I think of this scene, I always hear the words of my mother and father: "This money is for when you go to college."

My parents were already aware of my disability. I had never crawled or walked. I could not dress myself. I could sit unsupported if I was balanced just right; but if bumped (by a dog or another child) I would fall and there I would lie, calling for help, until someone picked me up. My parents were realistic about my limitations, of my weakness and difficulties in breathing. They dealt with the problems as they arose, but they did not dwell on the negative.

Instead, they watched constantly for things I was interested in and good at. I enjoyed art, and they kept me well supplied with paper, paints, markers, yarn, glue, and art books. I liked building things, and had a wide array of blocks and construction sets. Our home was full of music from the radio and the record player, and we all sang along. My mother read to me, and my father taught me my ABCs and numbers. I looked forward to the time when I would be old enough to go to school.

As I grew, my parents' words about the coin project came along with me. That simple sentence became a powerful expression of my family's dreams for my future. The goal at the time may have been college, but the message was broader in scope. I heard:

> Fly, Little One!
> Fly as high and as far and as fast
>   as your wings and your creativity can take you.
> The world is full of possibilities, and they are all there,
>   stretched out ahead for you to learn about and enjoy.

This year I will turn 40. I have long since graduated from college, gone to work, moved out on my own, and travelled from coast to coast. Yet the words, "This money is for when you go to college," are still a source of encouragement, just as they were when I sat on the floor, rolling coins.

WHEN KEVIN WAS BORN

Linda Meadows

When Kevin was born, the doctors said he wouldn't live through the night, or if he did, he would be a vegetable. Their way of comforting me was to say that I could have other children. I was furious with their insensitivity. I went home and cried for days.

It was a month or two before I first heard the term "cerebral palsy." My husband, Carl, and I received no information from the doctors about what this meant or what we should do. So I went to the library and read what I could, although there was not much available. Not knowing how to react, members of our family generally left us to ourselves. This was not ideal, but sometimes the alternative was worse. One day my mom was watching Kevin, and he choked when she was feeding him. She would have liked to continue watching him for us, but after that incident she was afraid. One of the other grandparents was even overheard telling someone that Carl and I should put Kevin in a home and go on with our lives. This hurt me a lot.

Fortunately, Carl and I had each grown up in neighborhoods where there was someone with a disability living down the street. Carl, in particular, saw a neighbor with cerebral palsy drive and go out with his girlfriend. Neither of us had any experience with people with disabilities close-up, but it gave us hope when we remembered these people we knew from a distance.

Carl and I were also in agreement that since Kevin was our child, we should be the ones taking care of him. He was our first, so everything was already new and overwhelming. Not knowing what to expect, we just took it one day at a time.

Kev grew and started attending a special school. Occasionally, someone would suggest that he might have mental retardation in addition to cerebral palsy. Carl and I resisted having this label put onto Kevin. We thought that people in the community might treat those with physical disabilities with encouragement and hope. They would be thought of as able to learn, and could achieve if given appropriate support. But we feared that the community would see no capacity, possibilities, or future for someone carrying the label of mental retardation. Expectations would be lower, and there would be a sense of "Why should we waste our time? They cannot learn anyway."

Already, people who were not close to Kevin seemed to underestimate him. Carl and I wondered why Kev spent several years of school struggling to learn colors instead of learning to read. The thinking was that he shouldn't progress to reading until he got his colors straight. Kevin never got very good at identifying colors, though. He is colorblind.

On the other hand, Kevin constantly surprised us with his powers of observance and understanding of mechanics. One day we were in a lighting store, and Carl and I walked around while Kev watched a man rewire a lamp. Kevin was trying to tell the man something, but his speech is difficult to understand. When we returned and the man asked me to translate, Kevin told him, "You wired it wrong." The man looked at the lamp, with the wire running through the various niches, and realized that he had missed one of the places the wire needed to go. He said, "Thank goodness you noticed that! I would have had to take it all apart again."

Another time, Kevin saw someone driving down our street with a special light on his trailer-hitch. He decided that he wanted to get the same thing for Carl for Father's Day. I tried and tried, but could not understand what Kevin had in mind. So together we went onto the Internet, and found the device he wanted. Then we were off to Pep Boys. Kevin was carrying the paper we had printed from the Internet. I went off to look for something else, and next thing I know here comes Kevin with the light he had wanted.

Labels can be misleading. We have friends who had a baby thirteen years ago. I remember when the father called me to let me know his son had been born. He said, "He has Down Syndrome. He has mental retardation." That is what the medical staff told him, that his child had mental retardation. Is it possible that they could be comparing this baby to other babies at one hour old, and already find him lacking in some way? What do newborn babies do besides eat and cry and sleep and need their diapers changed? Anyway, thirteen years later, this is a bright young man. He can outdo me on the computer, and he points out cars I could never identify.

Over the years, we have experienced many things because of Kevin. We have seen how preconceptions and labels place limits on people. We have fought, and watched others fight, for each individual to be valued for what he or she brings to the world. We have won some battles, and we have lost others. I try not to think about these things too much. Carl is the historian in our family. He remembers everything. But for me, reliving hurt feelings and lost opportunities only makes me depressed. I think it is best to leave the past in the past.

I look to the future. Thinking about the future is what gives me hope.

ALFRED FINDS A JOB

Pat Beeman and George Ducharme

Alfred carries the labels of multiple sclerosis and legal blindness. He moves around in a wheelchair. Upon first meeting Alfred, people might be tempted to focus on what he cannot do. Even so, his determination, great sense of humor, and knowledge of business computing, when made apparent, resulted in his acquisition of a job for himself.

We recognized Alfred's capacities and wanted to help him achieve his desire for employment. The first step was to connect him with a computer whiz who helped open some doors to the business community. When these open doors resulted in an interview with a major company, we brought Alfred to the interview and made ourselves available to interpret his difficult speech, but only if this became necessary. We made it a point to remain silent while Alfred impressed the three interviewers with his skills on a very complex computer program. At the end of the interview, Alfred shared the fact that he was legally blind. The interviewers were amazed. He got the job! His capacities and determination overshadowed his disabilities in the eyes of his new employers.

By offering the necessary support and resisting the opportunity to take over the process, Pat and George demonstrated the type of capacity seeking approach needed in One Candle Power. Capacity seeking may be forceful in the presence of injustice; but more often it is quiet, and discovered in the situation.

Guide to a Capacity Search

There is a growing body of literature about capacity-seeking geared toward the general public. Authors writing on self-help, career-planning, creativity, and community regeneration are touching on these themes. Writers such as Robert Bolles (*What Color Is Your Parachute?*), Sidney Parnes (*Visionizing*), Bernie Siegel (*Peace, Love and Healing*), and Robert Rodale (*Regenerating Community*) provide helpful guides for all people to sharpen their ability to find capacities in themselves and in others.

In the field of human services, we find the work of Beth Mount (*Personal Futures Planning*); John O'Brien and Connie Lyle (*The Five Essential Accomplishments*); and Jack Pearpoint, Marsha Forest, and Judith Snow (*PATH and The MAPS Process*) providing ways of discovering capacity with people who are labeled as having disabilities. These tools are helpful in searching for the opportunities that exist in every situation. To learn more about these resources as well as others, please see the section on Resources on page **183**.

A capacity search is simply the process of getting to know the focus person and building a description of the person that clearly displays the capacities and opportunities in his or her life. The process begins with an interview with the person, and perhaps a few other people who know the person well. If at all possible, the focus person should decide who will be there. He or she always has the final word, since the purpose of this exercise is to empower this person by listening to his or her preferences and dreams. The interview is like a treasure hunt. The facilitator is constantly looking for clues and opportunities to build on. Here is some material that would be helpful to include in the first interview.

BASIC INFORMATION

Background: What is the person's life story? What experiences from the past do we need to know about? What opportunities are present? What difficulties are present? What can we learn from the past?

Community and ethnic ties: What ties does this person have to the local community? Does he or she belong to any associations or groups in the local community? What other contacts are available? What ethnic or religious connections does this person have? What do these connections consist of? What opportunities are available in these ethnic or religious groups?

Family issues and concerns: What ties does the person have to immediate family? To the extended family? What resources and opportunities exist in the family? What are the concerns of the family about the future? What difficulties are experienced by the family? How are brothers and sisters doing? How is the health of older parents? What other dynamics do we need to know about?

Health and the body: What opportunities and barriers are present in the body? What limitations are imposed by health difficulties and physical disabilities? What are the barriers to community involvement because of accessibility or support needs? What are the opportunities for adaptive equipment?

COMMUNITY LIFE

Relationships: Who does the person spend the most time with on a daily and weekly basis? Who are other important people in this person's life? Who are the allies? Who might want to be involved in a circle of support?

Places: Where does this person go in the course of a day, a week, and a month? How many community places does the person use? How many human service settings? What places offer the most potential for increased participation? What places does this person want to move away from? What places provide the potential meeting space for a circle of support?

Choices: What choices does this person make? What choices are made by other people in his or her life? What activities require direct assistance from other people (i.e.: eating, using the bathroom, transportation)? How much autonomy does the person actually have? What opportunities are there to increase autonomy?

Barriers and opportunities to community acceptance: What personal characteristics does this person have that increase the likelihood of community acceptance? What characteristics might make community acceptance more difficult? Are there ways to reduce the impact of barriers? Are there ways to enhance positive qualities? How can the community address this person's need for respect?

PERSONAL PREFERENCES AND DESIRES

Personal preferences: What activities does this person enjoy most? When is this person most stimulated, engaged, and motivated? What activities and conditions are most frustrating? What conditions lead to boredom, anger, fear, or sadness? How can we increase positive experiences and decrease negative experiences?

Personal desires: What vision does this person have for his or her future? What dreams and hopes have gone unrecognized? What does this person want in life?

The Bottom Line: Recognizing Capacity

DO	DON'T
Look and listen long enough to find capacity	Concentrate on labels
Seek abilities not commonly valued in our society (i.e.: the ability to be present, the ability to bring people together)	Be put off by visible evidence of labels
Focus on the abilities of every person in the circle of support	Prejudge a person because of a label
Build on an individual's strengths	Deny disabilities, but do not dwell on them either
Focus on the unique opportunities of each association in a neighborhood or community.	Inadvertently damage people's reputation by begging for a chance to include or hire them

PLANNING A FUTURE

Several years ago, we experienced an apparent conflict between a person's vision and reality. When asked to describe his vision of the future, the young man said that he wanted to be an astronaut. Probably the same thought raced through the minds of everyone present: "How can someone labeled with mental retardation become an astronaut?" But we were not there to puncture his dream; we were there to walk with him toward its attainment. So off we went together.

Brainstorming produced the idea that this young man might get involved with the local planetarium. Connections were made, and soon he was working as an usher/ticket-taker, with all the fringe benefits like learning about the stars and meeting other people who were interested in space and space travel. When the group convened to consider the next step toward becoming an astronaut, the man said that he was happy at the planetarium, and that this was where he wanted to stay for now.

Traditionally, people without disabilities have been free to dream of where they want to live and what they want to do with their lives. Until recently, this basic right was denied to people with disabilities under the guise of "needing to be realistic."

Times have changed, and there is a growing recognition that all people benefit from pursuing their individual visions and interests. One way of transforming a dream into a reality is through a circle of support, a group of trusted friends who walk alongside someone as he or she pursues that dream. The dream gives purpose and focus to the circle. It gives circle members a flag to rally around.

In Connecticut, we have used the Personal Futures Planning process to help a circle clarify the vision and goals that the focus person has for his or her life. The group identifies the obstacles that prevent the accomplishment

> There is no power for change greater than a community discovering what it cares about.
>
> - Margaret Wheatley, Turning to One Another

of the goals, and develops strategies for overcoming these obstacles. By working together, the group can accomplish far more than any person working alone. The formation of a circle (whatever that looks like) must be emphasized because a vision without people working toward it is like a game plan with no team. Group action and commitment is what makes things happen.

A positive future is simply a summary of the experiences the focus person wants to have more of. The vision of the future is a summary of the opportunities and capacities the person has in his or her life. The vision is continually revised as the circle encounters new barriers and new opportunities.

The Steps of Personal Futures Planning, below, provide details which help groups identify goals and get started. The steps of this process are not as important as the dreams themselves. Several visions are provided to demonstrate the art of finding and shaping a dream.

The Steps of Personal Futures Planning

The details and sequence of the following steps will vary for each family or individual, but the process includes these components.

> The future belongs to those of us who believe in the beauty of our dreams.
>
> - Eleanor Roosevelt

Step 1: Identify Capacities

A. Map out relationships. Who is important to the focus person?

B. Map places. What are the patterns of life for the person now?

C. List personal preferences. What are the gifts the person has to offer in the life of the community?

D. Clarify personal dreams and desires. What goals does the person have?

Step 2: Identify a Planning Group

Using the "relationship map" developed in Step 1A, the focus person identifies the people he or she would like to ask to become part of the planning group. These people will meet on a regular basis to learn together how to make things happen for the focus person.

Step 3: Clarify a Personal Future

The focus person and his or her group work to clarify goals so they share a common vision of what they are trying to accomplish together.

Step 4: Identify Obstacles and Opportunities

Beginning with Step 1, obstacles, fears, and barriers to achieving the desired future are identified. These barriers offer a focus for problem-solving and for networking with other groups facing similar barriers.

Step 5: Generate Strategies

Circles meet regularly (usually about once every six weeks) to review what they have learned, celebrate what they have accomplished, and discuss new barriers and opportunities. They brainstorm to generate new strategies and directions for future activity.

Step 6: Make Commitments

Once the circle has reviewed the circumstances and done some brainstorming, members make commitments to work on specific strategies. Each member chooses the strategies that he or she has the energy to work on.

Step 7: Take Action

Group members take action. At first, many groups focus on learning more about community resources, program models, and barriers they are facing. As things progress, activities become more specific.

Step 8: Reflect on What the Group Is Learning

Every meeting is a time of reflection, but now and then (about twice a year) the group will meet to look again at "the big picture." It is good to refocus and to summarize recent accomplishments. This might be a good time for a party.

FIVE PEOPLE IMAGINE THE FUTURE

Judith Snow urges us to dream more than plan. Plans tend to become hardened: they lose the capacity to change. If you take the first step toward a dream, the dream will change as you go along. The dream will be changed by reality, but the dream will also change reality.

These five dreams were developed by people in 1987. The dreams and the actions taken to accomplish them changed over time. Community connections were made. Systems and policies were changed. Key to moving the process forward were the circles of support discussed on page 46. And as Judith Snow described, the dreams gradually changed shape as they came into contact with reality. Whether accomplished, modified, or abandoned, each dream took on a life of its own. Many gave rise to other dreams, which were based on what had already been learned.

CATHY lives in Wethersfield with her elderly mother. She works part-time as a writer and editor. Her images of the future include

1. Living in a HOUSING COOPERATIVE so that she does not have to live in a nursing home if something happens to her mother. Her home must include

   a. Personal Assistance – at least 6 hours a day

   b. Emergency medical support at home

   c. A good personal support system – everyone would live close together and she would know all of her neighbors

   d. An artist or writer's community in which all members could share their gifts

   e. A studio space that could be rented to artists outside the community

2. A FULL TIME JOB with a health plan and other benefits

3. Increased involvement in COMMUNITY LIFE, particularly artist and writer's associations

---

RAYMOND lives in a village that houses 100 people with disabilities. He works part-time for an insurance company. His images for his future include

1. A FULL TIME JOB with

    a. BENEFITS so he can get off of welfare

    b. The opportunity to CONTRIBUTE his skills and to use his Masters in Business Administration

2. A unit in a HOUSING COOPERATIVE, including

    a. A private room

    b. Support from personal assistants

    c. Easily accessible transportation

3. Increased involvement in COMMUNITY LIFE, particularly church, music, and the opportunity to RAISE A FAMILY

4. A more effective COMMUNICATION system

MATTHEW lives with his family. He is ten years old and attends public school in his community. His family envisions

1. RESPITE CARE and other forms of SUPPORT, such as

    a. RELIABLE, routine respite care on the weekends

    b. A family who knows Matthew well to provide backup support

    c. Respite care for EMERGENCIES

    d. An extended SUMMER CAMP program

    e. Low-interest loans for HOUSING ADAPTATIONS and MEDICAL SERVICES

2. RECREATION programs in the local community, such as

    a. Saturday morning programs at the local recreation department

    b. Horseback riding program

3. TRANSPORTATION so that Mom and Dad do not have to do all the driving

    a. During school for field trips

    b. To and from recreational activities

4. A stable HOME (not too far from the family home) so that Matthew can move out when he graduates from high school

KEVIN lives with his family and attends a special education facility outside of his community. He will finish high school in three years. His images of the future include

1. HIGH SCHOOL EXPERIENCES like

    a. Being in the regular high school

    b. Helping with a sports team

    c. Starting a T-shirt business with some other kids

    d. Learning to use computers

2. SUMMER PROGRAMS to expose him to the world of work, such as

    a. Summer jobs and work-study programs

    b. Art and music, summer theater programs

3. Increased involvement in COMMUNITY AND SOCIAL LIFE, including

    a. Places to go without Mom and Dad

    b. Belonging to community groups, kids' groups, and associations

4. A more effective COMMUNICATION system

JOHN lives with his family. He is at home most of the time, recovering from a serious accident he had seven years ago. John's family envisions

1. Family support, especially RESPITE CARE, that includes

    a. Reliable and trustworthy support people the family hires

    b. People who can lift John

    c. People who can understand him

    d. Respite support that is available for the weekends

2. DIRECT CONTROL of the aides and other helpers who come into the family home (6-8 different people come into the home every week; the family directly hires only one of these people). A VOUCHER PAYMENT system is needed which will enable the family to hire, train, and manage all support staff

3. Five-day-a-week PHYSICAL THERAPY for John

4. A COMMUNICATION SYSTEM that permits John to communicate more effectively

5. Always having a HOME for John, so that he never has to go into a nursing home

The notes from a personal futures session may take many forms. We find that a simple, colorful presentation on large paper, wherever possible, helps to focus attention on the vision being developed. Though not in color, the following page from my own dream is shown by way of illustration.

Reaching a vision is often a long and difficult journey. It helps to take others along with you to help with the process, and to share in the successes and failures. These traveling companions may be members of a circle of support, a technique described in the next section.

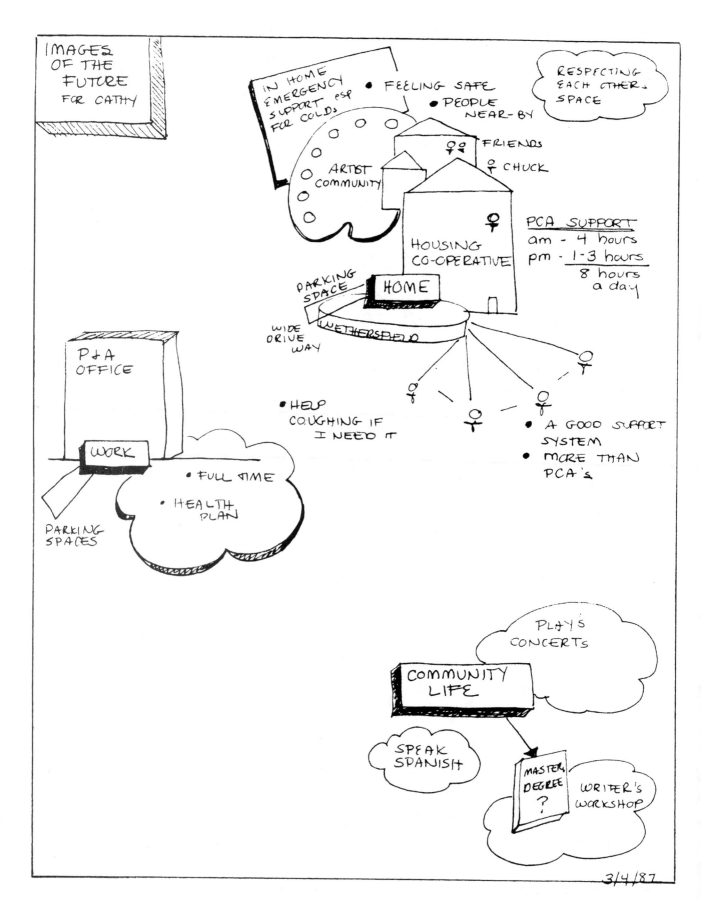

IMAGES
OF THE
FUTURE
FOR CATHY

IN HOME EMERGENCY SUPPORT esp FOR COLDS

● FEELING SAFE

● PEOPLE NEAR-BY

RESPECTING EACH OTHER, SPACE

ARTIST COMMUNITY

FRIENDS

CHUCK

HOUSING CO-OPERATIVE

PCA SUPPORT
am - 4 hours
pm - 1-3 hours
8 hours a day

PARKING SPACE

HOME

WETHERSFIELD

WIDE DRIVE WAY

P & A OFFICE

WORK

PARKING SPACES

● HELP COUGHING IF I NEED IT

● A GOOD SUPPORT SYSTEM
● MORE THAN PCA's

● FULL TIME

● HEALTH PLAN

PLAY'S CONCERTS

COMMUNITY LIFE

SPEAK SPANISH

MASTER DEGREE ?

WRITER'S WORKSHOP

3/4/87

Planning for the Future

Here is a letter describing the importance of planning for the future and engaging those around us to support us in our goals. The emphasis is on "creating great solutions by creating great stories, and then moving into them."

BREATHING LESSONS
David Wetherow

I wanted to share an e-mail exchange from one of the 'parent-to-parent' Internet mailing lists. A parent wrote:

> Today, I signed [my son] up on the waiting list for MR Waiver and group home or supportive living placement. The wait is about 10 years or so. I'm hoping that by the time he finishes high school, he can transition into adulthood and become more independent. Too many parents wait and wait, and when they seek these services, then they have to wait years and become very frustrated. Too often, young adults will regress if they are left home with nothing to do. For some reason, I thought of the clients I once served and got the urge to do it today. It's done :) A few of these clients had elderly parents in poor physical health who were trying to scramble to make arrangements only to be told of the waiting lists.

As a regular correspondent on the list, I wanted to address the notion that 'group home' might be a desirable direction to 'sign up for,' so I responded:

Dear M., I'm about to take some liberties with your story, but my experience has been that the way we create great solutions is to create great stories and then 'move into them.' I hope you receive this in the spirit in which I'm writing, with respect and admiration. You wrote:

> Today, I signed [my son] up on the waiting list for MR Waiver and group home or supportive living placement. The wait is about 10 years or so.

The important thing to remember (if I'm reading this correctly) is that what M. has done is to begin the process of establishing her son's entitlement to draw upon public resources when he comes 'of age.' She hasn't made any pre-determination about the shape of the specific services that she might purchase/engage with those resources (group home, supported living, etc.) - she's just set the wheels in motion for dollars to flow at the right time. (I would personally strongly encourage her to pursue the direction of supported interdependent living over a group home 'solution,' but that's my own experience and value base speaking.)

I'm hoping that by the time he finishes with high school, he can transition into adulthood and become more independent.

One of the things I'm sure that M. knows is that her son's 'independence' will be a blend of interdependence and self-determination. It will only be partially based on skills that he might acquire between now and the time he finishes high school. The real quality of his life will be anchored in established relationships with family, friends, allies, and champions - the heart of a living personal support network. Her work over the next five or ten years will be to seek out, invite and support those relationships.

Too many parents wait and wait and when they seek these services, then they have to wait years and become very frustrated. Too often, young adults will regress if they are left home with nothing to do.

M. understands that the service system has a very limited capacity to create good futures for our sons and daughters. At best, it can support and complement the work of community and family. At worst, it may neglect or abandon people, or provide stop-gap solutions that are uninspiring and unsatisfying.

On the other hand, if M. does a good job of engaging her son's community way ahead of time, friends, extended family members, church partners, colleagues from work, etc. can work creatively to offer employment opportunities (beginning with after-school and summer jobs), learn about his interests and gifts, and make sustaining commitments to her son's employment and contribution to the community.

For some reason, I thought of the clients I once served and got the urge to do it today. It's done :) A few of these clients had elderly parents in poor physical health who were trying to scramble to make arrangements only to be told of the waiting lists.

M. is absolutely on target here. It is essential for families to gather their community around them and in a spirit of companionship begin to create plans, invite commitments, and take action. The amazing thing is how strongly the community will respond when we share our story, and share our dreams.

By far, the best guide for doing this work is Al Etmanski's book, A Good Life, available at http://www.agoodlife.org. It's one of the best investments a family can make, whether their child is 10, or 20, or 40. If a family can't afford the book, the local ARC, parent organization or public library certainly can, and one can always encourage them to add it to their collection.

M. said, "I did it…" - and she's done the right thing. There's a lot of creative work ahead, but she's putting the foundation pieces into place. Fair winds!
Cheers,
David

P.S. We've been up for six nights trying to keep Amber breathing, so I'm sorry if this is a bit rough around the edges.

One of the other list members was kind enough to respond:

Dave, I hope Amber is better. I will be keeping you and your daughter in my thoughts. Take care – all your posts are wonderful and give me much to think about. Please let us know if Amber is breathing better.

I responded:
Thanks P. (and others who took the time to express the same hope).
We'll get there. Actually, this is the first time in fifteen years that Amber has had a serious lung infection, which is a little miracle considering how much she struggles with aspiration and what a trial it is for her to eat and drink. Faye does this amazing 'slow dance' with her every mealtime—positioning every spoonful of food, managing textures, etc.

Recently, it's taken two of us to help her through most meals, one feeding her and helping her position her mouth and chin, the other holding her arms up and gently trying to overcome the reflex extensions.

Sometimes just tipping her wrist forwards a bit allows her hand/arm/shoulder to relax for a few seconds—enough for one swallow.

All of this keeps me reminded that 'quality' is in the moments, that companionship is paramount, and that as we begin to think about expanding the family circle, what we're looking for is the possibility of inviting other people in who will see our kids the way we do, operate with the same integrity and resourcefulness, and find their part in the 'slow dance.'

We've done some thinking about this over the last several years. Last month, when we were doing a workshop, Faye was talking about these qualities and I was scrambling to create a graphic that portrayed what she was saying. For twenty years, we've been working on supports that were based on the idea of 'Moving forward from (actually with) the family model,' as opposed to 'Moving backwards from the institutional model.' The pattern is an initial attempt at depicting what families really do for their kids - all of their kids.

We share our lives—submit our lives to our children. What we really yearn for is to find other people whom we can draw into the family circle, who might share this journey with us and with our kids. This is what I'm talking about when I mention the idea of 'interdependent living'—moving forward from (and with) the family.

We've been observing the service system for longer than I care to think about, and we've been involved in over a hundred formal evaluations of services of all kinds. The observed reality is that 'services' will not and cannot do these things for our kids. But the great possibility is that, as families, we can invite and support relationships that will offer these things and will deliver them over the long haul.

In this pattern, the role of the State changes from that of service provider to one of financing the solutions that families and friends create together. In this pattern, the organizations that we think of as 'agencies' play a very different role: they move from 'service delivery' (where your child's life is no longer your own, or his own) to encouraging and supporting the work that the young person, the family and faithful companions are doing together.

This isn't a fantasy. In British Columbia, Vela Microboard Association has involved seven hundred friends and family members in creating and sustaining individualized solutions for a hundred and fifty men and women with disabilities (some of whom have extremely challenging disabilities indeed). The State's role is to provide financing, not 'services.' Vela is a well-designed small agency that helps those families and friends get organized and stay on track, and their work has been going on for over ten years. Currently, Faye and I are supporting the emergence of similar projects in Tennessee and Ontario.

When M. says "I really hope supportive living will work for him," I want to point out to her that supportive living is working for him now! Living with your family is supportive living.

What works in M's son's life—what allows his life to 'work,' what allows him to be successful right now—is that her son is living in a context of relationship, devotion, love, respect, and a constantly evolving 'slow dance.' Now the work is to expand the number of people who are involved in that dance, to invite commitment, to practice together, so that if and when [her son] leaves his family home, what he experiences is just 'changing partners' and continuing the dance with people in whom he already has confidence and who have confidence in him. M. and her husband can continue their dance, and watch with delight as their son continues his.

If you put it together right, it literally cannot fail. Because it's not built on 'skills;' it's built on companionship and devotion and continuous adaptation. It's not a 'program' that somebody can 'fail;' it's a dance.

Very early in our work, we helped Nicola and Ted Schaefer create a home for their daughter Catherine that was very much like her original family home. Kate went from living with her parents and brothers to living with housemates who Nicola recruited, trained and supported (with the long-run assistance of a small cooperative agency that we created together, with Kate and her mom as the first members). Over the following fifteen years, there have been a lot of changes - new housemates, the family sometimes dancing close, sometimes farther away, big swings in Catherine's health, changes in thinking about what 'daytime' should look like - new steps in the dance.

This is supported living at its best. When Catherine's health changed, it did not fail—something about the dance changed. When Kate became dismally unhappy with what was going on during the day, it did not fail—

something about the dance changed. When a partner forgot what he or she was there for, it did not fail—another partner entered the dance. Now the thing that I haven't told you yet is that Catherine is massively disabled ... the whole nine yards. But this young woman, who has a list of disabilities as long as your arm, has been living in her own home for over fifteen years—because it was built on the right premise.

The premise was simply moving forward from (and with) the family. Nicola and Ted said, "What Catherine has now is great!", and then they asked, "What would this look like in the next phase of her life?" They were brave and creative about inviting people in. They were innovative about re-working the relationships between Catherine, family, government, 'agency,' and life-sharing companions.

Has it always been smooth? Well, as Charles Shultz's Charlie Brown reminds us, "Grief is a Constant." Look at what the last two weeks has been like for Amber and us. This week's dance has us awake at three in the morning. This week's dance even had some scary moments. But look! There's a little bit of light coming back into her eyes. A trace of humour is flickering across her face. And as I left her room a few minutes ago to continue writing this letter, she turned and said, "Welcome!" (actually, 'wo-cum,' which we know really means 'thank you').

Yes, she's breathing better, just a little bit at a time. And so are we.
Love,
David

David and Faye Wetherow share their lives with an adopted daughter who has complex mobility and communication challenges. They have long been involved in innovative service development, creative facilitation and community-building.

911 Terrien Way
Parksville, BC V9P1T2 CANADA
Phone: 250 248-2531
Fax: 250 248-2685
http://www.community-works.net
wetherow@shaw.ca

BUILDING CIRCLES

> *A little boy, in the presence of his father,*
> *was trying to move a rock -- almost as big as he was!*
>
> *Though he was straining and groaning,*
> *it was simply too much for him and he gave up,*
> *all out of breath and exhausted.*
>
> *"You weren't using all your strength," commented the father.*
> *"Oh yes I was," the boy insisted,*
> *frustrated and disappointed in himself.*
>
> *"Oh, but you weren't," was the father's simple reply.*
> *"You didn't ask me to help you!"**

Contrary to popular belief, independence is usually not achieved by an "I'm going to do it all by myself" attitude. The key is to establish and nurture relationships in which everyone is able to do something for someone else. Circles of support focus the attention and abilities of a natural network (such as family, friends, and neighbors) on accomplishing a particular goal. Individual strengths and talents are multiplied as circle members join forces. Likewise, weaknesses become less significant because of the combined abilities of the group.

A circle may be a place for support, but its real purpose is action. It is a place for hard work. As people meet in a spirit of care and concern for another, they also learn a great deal as they work together to make the vision or goal happen. The circle builds a group of people who are ready to do whatever it takes – open doors, change systems – whatever they can do to bring the vision closer to reality.

---

*   From *Take a Break – Everybody Needs One!: Calls to Worship* by Ernst Nussmann, 1997, page 25. Used by permission from CSS Publishing Company, 517 S. Main Street, P.O. Box 4503, Lima, Ohio 45802-4503.

BIRTH OF THE JOSHUA COMMITTEE
Jack Pearpoint*

On that fateful morning, someone eventually materialized and got Judith up. She drove her chair over to her friend Peter Dill's office. She uttered a few words, "I can't do it any more..." Then Judith stopped talking. For many of us, this might increase the clarity of our communication. For Judith, it meant no communication. She had given up. She just couldn't manage any more. She knew what the system's response would be – reinstitutionalization. Consciously she had decided she would rather die. But in a last desperate flailing for help, she drove to Peter's office. Later she recalled hoping that Peter would understand she was at wits end. If her friends wanted her to live, they would have to figure it out. She couldn't do it alone any more.

Peter figured that much out. He called Marsha. Marsha called me and a van, and in the afternoon, Judith was transported to our house. Marsha and I made a cozy little recovery room upstairs. I carried Judith up and left her to rest. Shaunee, our yellow labrador had a long standing licking relationship with Judith. They didn't need speech. Shaunee, sensing Judith's trauma, nuzzled in and lick-washed her hands and face. Some people might have been offended. For Judith, it was maternal healing. Just like a dog to do what we humans couldn't.

Meanwhile, we phoned Judith's friends and called an emergency meeting in our living room that night. There were fourteen people. Judith didn't want to come down, or even send a message. It was up to us.

We all had to decide if we wanted Judith in the world – and if so, how we were going to make that happen. Even in a few hours of providing attendant care, we had learned that this was not a task you just slipped into a busy day. It was a busy day in its own right. The first decision was self-evident. People had come because they were committed to Judith

* This story appears in the book *From Behind the Piano* as a chapter titled, "Judith Collapsed..." It has been reprinted with the permission of the author. The Joshua Committee paved the way for many other circles of support. For information about ordering this book and other excellent materials from Inclusion Press, please look in the Part 4: Resources.

being in the world with us. How? What was needed? What would we do? We were all a bit frantic. But within the group, we formed natural interest teams to tackle various issues.

- ♦ Someone needed to be sure that Judith was talked back from the brink of suicidal stress. Peter volunteered to be the lead person and organize others to support him.
- ♦ Judith would need a place to live. The group from York University, led by Marsha and Peter, agreed to pull out all the stops to try and get decent housing on campus immediately.
- ♦ Attendant care translated into dual crises – personnel and money. Several of the group worked out shifts on the spot to cover the following two weeks. Peter Dill recruited two of his colleagues from the National Institute on Mental Retardation (NIMR) [now the Canadian Association for Community Living – CACL]. Peter Clutterbuck and I agreed to intensify our lobbying for money for attendant care. We were already convinced from this most recent collapse that a totally voluntary system was stop-gap at best. Sandy Gray agreed to coordinate the volunteer attendants, in the hope that we would find a budget before volunteers burned out.

That weekend, in the midst of the chaos, Marsha and I went to Guelph for a conference. In spite of the crisis, we were confident that all was in hand, and Judith was secure at our house. I had forgotten about our leaving. Judith recalled the tension very quickly. She thought we were abandoning her. She didn't know us well enough to understand that this was normal for us. We weren't abandoning – just busy. We of course had no notion of the extent of Judith's fear of abandonment. We hadn't really understood it at West Park when her parents lectured at us. Judith never mentioned it. How could we have understood? So that weekend, in the midst of a survival crisis, we laid the seeds for the next crisis of confidence. Judith did the only thing she could. She judged us on the basis of a life long experience of abandonment. We didn't even see the problem. It's hard to understand life from someone else's shoes.

Within two weeks, there was a kind of stability in Judith's life. Sandy Gray undertook the round-the-clock coordination of attendant care.

Peter and Marsha got the University to allocate a student apartment for Judith. Peter Dill's personal support was bringing Judith back into voice. Peter Clutterbuck and I worked on budgets and proposals. There was movement within the Ministry of Community & Social Services (COMSOC) regarding funding. The problems weren't all solved, but we had begun to learn how to work together. Although we didn't know it yet, the Joshua Committee was at work.

What Is a Circle of Support?

A circle of support is a group of people who agree to meet on a regular basis to assist the focus person to accomplish personal visions or goals. The individual is unable to reach these goals working alone, perhaps because of a disability, or obstacles related to the disability. So he or she invites a number of people to work together to blaze a path to new opportunities. Circle members provide support to the focus person and take action on his or her behalf.

The members of a circle of support are usually friends, family members, co-workers, neighbors, congregation members, and sometimes service providers. The majority of people in a circle of support are not paid to be there. They are involved because they care about the person and have made a commitment to work together to make the person's life better. Circles in no way exclude paid providers of human services. Service providers can be an essential resource to a circle of support. Still, the majority of circle members are typical community members who are there just because they care.

When the majority of people in a circle of support are paid human service workers, we prefer to call this a "person-centered team." These teams also work toward a positive future for the focus person, but the characteristics of this team are different from those of a community-based circle of support (see comparison on pages 65-68).

Four Steps to Building a Circle

1. FOCUS on an individual; GENERATE a vision

A vision of what the individual wants will help set guidelines and plan strategies. Do not take on too much at once. The overall vision may be ambitious (i.e.: moving out and getting a job); but starting small and ensuring positive results will allow more difficult steps to be approached with confidence and a history of working together as a group. Knowing the vision will help everyone stay centered when barriers get in the way. Prepare a road map: know where you are starting, where you are going, how you will get there, when, and with whom.

Some hints for creating a vision:

♦ Instead of knocking ideas, listen to the desires of the individual. Build on the things he or she says. Listening to feelings. Feelings are neither right nor wrong. They just are.

♦ Assist the individual to be "capacity seeking:" to see the best in oneself and in others.

♦ Look at the person's gifts and contributions to make the vision come alive.

♦ Consider what the realistic barriers are.

♦ How can the community become part of removing those barriers and making the vision real?

♦ Don't expect things to happen overnight.

♦ Every person has a unique contribution to make. Let each person share his or her gifts with the group. These gifts are as various and as numerous as those who possess them.

2. EMPOWER the focus person or family; learn what they see as a vision and work with them to achieve it

Don't tell them what is right for them or for their child.

Help them to see THEIR CAPACITIES and work toward the goal with them.

Get them as close to the dream as possible.

Remember that EMPOWERMENT STARTS FROM THE INSIDE. It does not work from outside in. People sometimes short-circuit the process for others by trying to do the task of self-empowerment for them. We tend to think automatically of doing something for the other person, and do not consider that the person can do something with and for us as well.

Don't give the impression that professionals have all the answers.

3. WORK WITH interested friends, family, and individuals who care

Have the focus person or focus family invite family members, friends, and neighbors to become part of the circle of support.

Look for the "gifts" of the people within the circle.

View different ideas as ways to discover more and see new solutions to a problem.

Develop strategies to overcome the obstacles and BRING THE VISION TO LIFE for the individual or family.

Certain people in the circle may be able to act as a "bridge" into associations and activities in the community for the focus person or family. Identify these people and find ways for them to use this opportunity.

4. FIND CONNECTIONS within existing family, friends, neighbors, and community resources. Look to everyone for ways to get more involved in community.

Where do relatives and friends work? What clubs do they belong to? Are they involved in religious groups, such as churches? How might they get you in the door?

Who are they? Who are their families? What are their particular needs and interests?

Look through local newspapers and newsletters to find ways to meet the challenges to reaching each person's vision.

But How Does It Actually Work?

A circle of support is formed when the focus person, or in some cases his or her spokesperson, asks for help from the people they know. They ask people if they are willing to collaborate on reaching a common goal. It is important to collect some background information, perhaps developing a Personal Futures Plan to lend structure to the process. Creating a relationship map is part of Personal Futures Planning, and is simply a drawing of the people who are important to the focus person.

After the relationship map is complete and a Futures Plan has been developed, ask the focus person to choose who he or she would like to invite to the initial meeting. If people need help to extend the invitation, offer to assist them. People have invited from five to 25 people to their first circle meeting. On the next page is a relationship map and a list of important places in someone's life (in this case, mine).

We have found that circle members tend to fall into three categories of involvement. A small group often becomes the core of the circle. Members of this core group usually attend all circle meetings, and they may also work extra hard between meetings to carry out tasks that will move the process forward. The second group of circle members may be committed to the focus person and the vision, but be less involved in the process. They may come to some circle meetings and lend a hand now and then. Around the edges of the circle, there may be resource people who come to a circle meeting only once. This is a third layer of support. These might include a minister, a Town Council member, or a distant relative. They want to be kept informed, and we know we can count on them if their help is needed, but they are not usually available on a day-to-day basis.

> # Observations
> ## From Circle Members and Circle Builders
>
> The circle building process is "elliptical." By elliptical I mean that the path a circle takes is not a straight line, that at times we move away from the dream or vision we are searching for as surely as we move back again toward it in another direction. No matter how intently we set upon the path, there are bound to be detours and dry places, stretches of darkness we fear we might never emerge from. Such doubts and distractions are not unusual. In fact, these difficulties are built into the very process of our growth together as a circle supporting the vision for an individual.
>
> Pat Beeman

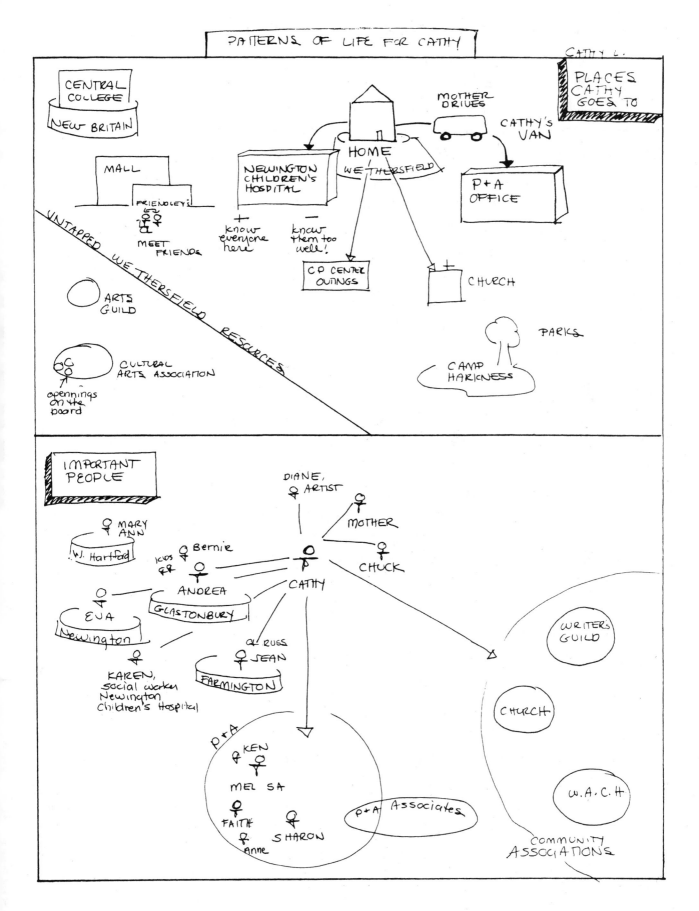

PATTERNS OF LIFE FOR CATHY

When and Where Do Circles of Support Meet?

Meeting location is essential to supporting the participation of circle members. Circles typically meet in people's living rooms, meeting rooms at the local church or library, restaurants or diners, or other spaces that make it convenient for people to attend. If the focus person or a circle member need a space that is wheelchair accessible, look for spaces that meet that criterion. As much as possible, circles should meet in community settings and not in conference rooms at human service agencies.

Meeting times are based on individual preference. Circles often meet in the evening or on weekends because the majority of people have daytime commitments. There may be occasions, however, when people would prefer to meet during the day, and there is nothing wrong with this. Do whatever works. Keep it informal. Meetings have a set format, but they are fun and intense at the same time. People often prepare snacks, and we celebrate a lot as part of these meetings. Children may attend, and pets can also liven things up. We laugh a lot. We struggle together as we work our way through the obstacles people face, and learn the complexities of each situation. The actual meeting takes about two hours. People often stay and chat afterward.

Circles may meet monthly. Many meet every six weeks. Some circles working on complicated issues may have subcommittee (sometimes called "semicircle") meetings to accomplish things in between the larger meetings. The whole process can be intense, requiring many brainstorming sessions, phone calls, and excursions. Depending on what the group is working on, some circles may not meet during the summer.

Again, everything hinges on the focus person, how quickly he or she wants to progress, and the availability of circle members. No two groups ever function alike.

> As a result of my circle of support, I am more confident in making some waves rather than being status quo about a situation I would like to change.
>
> Raymond Kilroy

What Happens During a Circle Meeting?

A facilitator is essential to an effective circle meeting. The facilitator is someone who agrees to conduct the meeting by beginning the activities, keeping a record of the discussion, summarizing the ideas generated, and helping people make commitments to action. The facilitator may be the person with the dream, or it may be a friend or someone brought in from outside to get things started. It is important that the facilitator understand the person's vision, preferences, and social network.

The first time a circle meets, the objectives are to get everyone acquainted with one another and with the vision the group will pursue. The facilitator has already met with the focus person to get a sense of themes in the person's life, to identify his or her goals, and to gain an understanding of the opportunities and obstacles facing the person. Usually, this process is drawn on large sheets of paper. We call this a "graphic future" because it provides diagrams and pictures of a person's life.

The facilitator reviews the graphic future with members of the group by putting the paper up on the wall or by handing out smaller drawings. It is important to describe the role of a circle of support, and to explain the process so people do not feel lost. The best way is by telling stories of other circles and how they worked. The rest of the meeting is spent brainstorming strategies to bring a vision into reality. Identify which part of the vision to focus on first: looking for an apartment or planning supports, for example. Don't try to do everything at once.

In the last ten minutes of the meeting, the facilitator goes over all the strategies that have been suggested. Five to ten action items with commitments are the result of a productive meeting. The focus person decides which of these are worth pursuing (all ideas are welcome, but some may seem more appropriate than others). Then circle members have the opportunity to make

> The work is more an art than a science. The solution is as likely to come from your imagination as from your rational mind. It's not a matter of designing programs but of creating visions; not of following protocols but fulfilling dreams. And believing in those dreams; believing that a woman who has been isolated could still have friends, or that a man whose life had been controlled could still escape and be free. Trusting that kind of vision means learning to hope.
>
> *The Gift of Hospitality*
> Mary O'Connell

commitments to act on these strategies. It is important not to overload people, but if each circle member takes one or two assignments, this is usually manageable. The group chooses a time and place to meet again, and then the meeting adjourns. Below is a summary of the steps for a first meeting.

> The gifts of each person participating in a circle can make a difference. It is possible for anyone to contribute to achieving a vision.
>
> George Ducharme

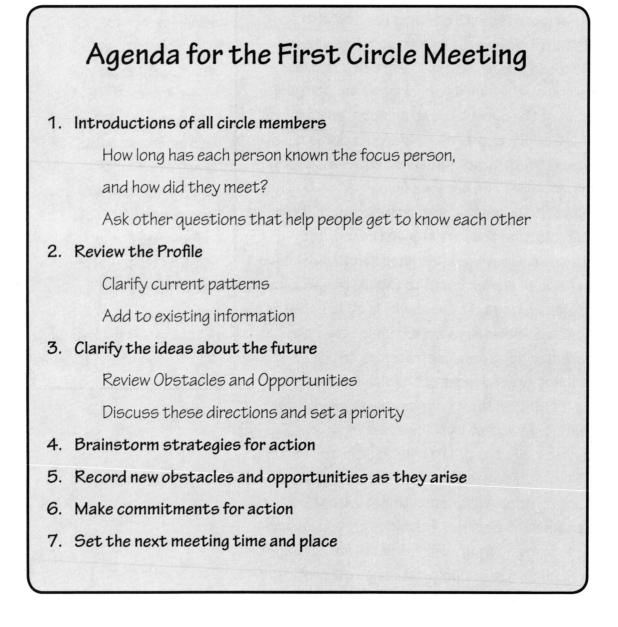

Agenda for the First Circle Meeting

1. **Introductions of all circle members**

    How long has each person known the focus person,

    and how did they meet?

    Ask other questions that help people get to know each other

2. **Review the Profile**

    Clarify current patterns

    Add to existing information

3. **Clarify the ideas about the future**

    Review Obstacles and Opportunities

    Discuss these directions and set a priority

4. **Brainstorm strategies for action**

5. **Record new obstacles and opportunities as they arise**

6. **Make commitments for action**

7. **Set the next meeting time and place**

The first few meetings are a time of reflection and clarification, while followup meetings provide an ongoing opportunity to strategize. Initial meetings are especially revealing because circle members become fully aware of the barriers faced by the person with a disability, often for the first time. This first meeting is critical because it defines the focus and creates solidarity and commitment from participants.

The followup meetings are equally important, but in a different way. The facilitator begins by reviewing the priorities from the last meeting. Members then share their activities, frustrations, and accomplishments. Actions of the group are recorded in two ways: "Things that Work" (new opportunities and positive findings) and "Things that Don't Work" (new barriers and negative findings).

For an example, see the next page.

After discussing how the activities turned out, the group strategizes, members make commitments to carry out the next set of activities, another meeting is planned, and the process begins again.

Agenda for Follow Up Meetings

1. **Review commitments from last meeting**

2. **Members report on progress**

    Information is sorted into new opportunities and new obstacles

3. **Brainstorm new strategies**

4. **Record obstacles and opportunities as they arise**

5. **Make commitments to action**

6. **Set next meeting time and place**

Things That Work	Things That Don't Work
Engaging, enjoyable, motivating:	**Frustrating, upsetting, boring:**
<ul><li>Being a writer.</li><li>Being with people.</li><li>Disability issues including participating in advocacy groups, writing, & public speaking.</li><li>Politics, politics! Public speaking.</li><li>Having a slow & flexible pace.</li><li>Going to meetings, conferences, & places.</li><li>The job a Protection & Advocacy.</li><li>Relatively secure work with benefits.</li><li>Room to grow and change.</li><li>A job with insurance, or have a Medicare and Blue Cross supplement (one or the other).</li><li>Having a good van, & increasing the numbers of people who can drive the van.</li></ul>	<ul><li>Having weak lungs; I have to have help if I need to cough.</li><li>I can do a lot, but not very fast. For example, it takes about 2 hours to eat.</li><li>I have to remember and plan to eat. It takes so long and I'd rather be doing other things..</li><li>When everything takes a long time, people often don't understand.</li><li>Not having parking spaces at home or at work.</li></ul>
Things That Will Help: **Opportunities**	**Obstacles and Fears:**
<ul><li>The housing co-operative idea.</li><li>Dave Wetherow's vision of an artist's co-operative.</li><li>Ed Preneta is looking into government loans for co-ops.</li><li>Sarah Page is becoming an expert on co-opseratives</li><li>Cathy has received the PACA program from DHR that pays $7300 per years.</li><li>P and A is attempting to get Cathy a full time job with benefits.</li><li>George knows people in the artist/writer community.</li><li>Having a good job at P and A.</li><li>Cathy has Medicare and SSDI tied to father's work record.</li><li>Blue Cross Supplement.</li></ul>	<ul><li>The co-op idea is very complex. How do we do it? How do we get the money?</li><li>Personal Care Attendant costs, building trust & accountability; learning how to manage PCA's.</li><li>If anything happens to my mom: no where to go.</li><li>DHR PCA program is not enough - we need about $18,000 a year.</li><li>If Cathy lost her job, or couldn't work, she would lose the PCA support.</li><li>If Cathy gets sick, she needs a lot of help. A cold can put her out of work for two weeks.</li><li>Will have to have insurance to pay for in-home nursing care if she gets sick.</li><li>The current P and A contract arrangement enables Cathy to keep Medicare. Consequently, it is a small contract, with low pay.</li><li>Cathy faces the possibility of becoming more dependent over time.</li><li>If she lost father's SSDI benefits, work record too short to get back on.</li><li>Using community medical resources is hard.</li><li>If we use a 3 family house to create a co-op, we would have a problem with parking for 6 cars and those of guests and PCA's.</li><li>Someone has to drive the van to work.</li></ul>

What Is the Circle "Accomplishing"?

The actual accomplishments of each circle of support vary greatly, in the same way that circle composition, meeting style, and goals vary from one situation to another. Some circles are able to solve problems right away just by having extra support and a focused approach. Most circles, however, work on complex issues that take a long time to change. Some concentrate on integrating children into the public school system; this requires constant collaboration with the school, and the need to continually arrive at creative solutions. Other circles have the objective of finding housing options so people can move out on their own. Sometimes these options do not exist yet, or if they do, there may be financial obstacles or accessibility barriers standing between the person and his or her goal. Along with the need for housing, employment, or educational opportunities there may be the additional issue of supports. Again, people may need formalized services that do not yet exist in the service system. They must then work at a policy level to change the system (see "Changing Systems," page 86).

Focus people and circle members certainly become discouraged at times. Circles go through periods of great struggle and long stretches of hard work when progress is difficult to see. Often, these challenging periods are followed by "breakthroughs," and for a while positive outcomes may occur at a rapid rate. Then because of these changes, people are faced with new sets of problems. In other words, "circles have cycles." Simply because everything takes so long and requires so much effort, we look for small victories along the way. We try to find ways to renew the vision and re-energize the work of the group.

Kevin's story reflects the outcomes of an ongoing process of struggle and celebration. Next, my brief essay describes the simple but profound change the circle process made in my own life. Finally, Debbie's story shows that people without disabilities can also benefit from a circle of support, and that occasionally a dream can be reached with just one or two meetings.

KEVIN'S CIRCLE

Based on a presentation by Linda and Kevin Meadows[*]

Kevin attended a hospital school in a suburb of Hartford for 13 years. But because the students all came from different towns, they tended to scatter as soon as school was out. So Kevin never had the opportunity to make friends or to form any lasting relationships at this school.

After awhile we had to make a move, so we sent Kevin to another special school in a small city closer to our home. But again, the kids were bused in from all over, and he couldn't make any friends.

When we started our circle, we invited some close friends who had kids, and asked the kids what they thought Kevin needed. Our younger son, Jason, said that if Kevin thought his school was rough, he ought to try going to a regular school. All the kids agreed that Kevin should go to our local high school.

At our meetings, the kids told us who the best teachers were, and figured out who could help Kevin with different things during the school day. The school psychologist was on our side, and he took down all their ideas. At first we were only able to get Kevin into the local high school once a semester. But when it was time for the PPT (Pupil/Parent/Teacher meeting), we invited so many people that we almost couldn't get everyone into the room. Students spoke about how good it would be to have Kevin in school with them, and explained how they thought it could work. By now, not only the psychologist but all the special ed and regular ed teachers, administrators, and other team members were becoming enthusiastic.

Kev attended the local high school full time for two years, and he worked above the capacity anyone thought he had. He made friends on the basketball team, so he was always going to games. He also joined Peer Leadership, an afterschool club involved in community service.

People want to help if you just tell them how. We never could have done this without the support of our friends.

---

[*]   This story is adapted from *The P & A Update*, Summer, 1988, and is based on a presentation by the Meadows family at "One Candle Power," an introduction to the circle process, held on May 11, 1988.

REPLACING "I AND ME" WITH "WE AND US"
Cathy Ludlum

A strange thing happened the first time I was asked to talk about the circle. I wrote a speech that described my long search for a housing situation; how I tried to find a way to afford 24 hours a day of personal assistance; how I seriously considered moving to a segregated community in another part of the country; how I even attempted to start a group home for people with physical disabilities. Although I put huge amounts of energy and optimism into these projects, in the end I was no better off than I had been before.

Then I wrote about the friends and colleagues who became my circle. Common interests emerged when little clusters of people formed to discuss cooking, computers, kids, and civil rights. Phone numbers were exchanged and lunches planned. Soon, the circle was no longer *my* circle, but a community of friends where everyone could benefit. Together we tackled the conditions which prevented me from living independently and we saw progress.

When I read what I had written, I realized that I had gotten nowhere as long as I struggled alone. Only when "I and me" were replaced by "we and us" did the dream start to look attainable. Even when things get bogged down, as they inevitably do, we give each other support and encouragement, and keep on looking for the creative answers we can only find as a community of friends.

CIRCLES ARE FOR EVERYONE
Debbie Barisano

I needed to make a very difficult decision. I was in college, with only five courses left before I earned my Associate Degree in the Disability Specialist Program at Manchester [Connecticut] Community College. There were obstacles to me finishing my degree, and I could not see any way around them.

I had been working in the disability field as a personal assistant for about one year. Although I was excited about my job, the pay was low. I was putting in about 45 hours a week, and I was already struggling to pay my bills. To graduate, I was required to complete two semesters with 120 internship hours per semester. Yet I could not reduce my paid employment and still manage my expenses.

How could I possibly fulfill the responsibilities of an internship while still working over 40 hours a week as a personal assistant? On top of all that, how could I fit in the last few classes and the necessary coursework? Some of the classes were only offered at odd times when I would normally be working. Would having an Associate Degree really get me anywhere in terms of my future? How could I get past these obstacles? Should I quit school? These were all questions that needed to be answered before I could make an informed decision. In addition, with the real-life experience I was gaining in my job, the college courses I had once enjoyed did not seem as interesting anymore.

In my disability courses I had learned about circles of support, which were sometimes used by people with disabilities to talk out issues and solve problems. I did not have a disability, but why wouldn't this work for me? I decided to form my own circle to help me with this decision. I knew that if I continued in school, I would need the support of friends to keep me motivated and to help with some of the obstacles. I invited my employers, the director of my college program, and two friends to be in my circle.

We met one evening in my employer's living room. I described my goals and dreams for the future, the work needed to finish college, and the roadblocks I perceived. It was amazing! We brainstormed creative ways that I could do my internship without losing any time from work. A friend gave me a new perspective about how not to be bored while taking my remaining college courses. He suggested that I look at it as an opportunity to teach other students about people with disabilities. It was a very motivational meeting! At the end of the evening, all I could see were opportunities, and I felt a new excitement toward finishing my degree. My circle only met once, but the support of the circle has been there ever since.

My two internship semesters were busy but successful, and I ultimately did finish school. I was the Salutatorian of my class and was awarded honors for my work in the disability field. Many of my circle members were at the awards ceremony and at graduation. They reminded me that I had almost quit school. We all agreed that the circle meeting was a turning point, and shared our happiness that I had finished my degree.

Circles of support may have begun around people with disabilities, but there is no reason why everyone cannot use this good idea.

How Are Circles of Support
Different from Other Planning Groups?

Planning futures for people has become fashionable in the disability field. Many human service workers are seeking to improve the individual planning process so that people's plans reflect their preferences and interests. They are working to change human service organizations to be more supportive of life experiences chosen by the focus person and people who know his or her dreams the best. We refer to these efforts as "person-centered planning," and strongly support continued movement in this direction.

Building circles, however, is a very different process from other types of individual planning in human services. A circle of support forms and operates totally in the interest of the focus person. The focus person and/or a trusted spokesperson determine every aspect of the circle including membership, setting, image of the future, and frequency of meetings. The circle does not belong to "the system." The circle is located in the local community and depends on that community for its effectiveness.

We have provided two forms of comparison to illustrate the differences between various types of planning. The first compares traditional (interdisciplinary team) planning, person-centered planning, and circles of support. A second is a description of what is and what is not a circle of support.

A Comparison of Three Types of Planning for People with Disabilities and Elders

Beth Mount

Traditional Planning	Person-Centered Teams	Circles of Support
Purpose of the Planning Meeting:		
To coordinate services across disciplinary lines. To clarify staff roles in the implementation of programs.	To establish a common vision for all staff. To discover information needed to focus organizational change.	To establish and support a personal vision for an individual. To build community support and action on behalf of the focus person.
Composition of the Team:		
Professionals and specialists.	Professionals and direct service workers. May include focus person and family.	Focus person, his or her spokesperson, family, friends, and associates. May include some human service workers.
Where Does the Group Meet?		
Conference room in a human service agency or similar setting: centralized site.	Human service setting close to direct service workers (group home, sheltered workshop): decentralized site.	Community setting (living room, church meeting room, library conference room): places close to where circle members live.
How Often Does the Group Meet?		
Once a year with quarterly reviews.	Major investment in initial sessions. Quarterly or monthly reviews.	Every 4-6 weeks, possibly with subcommittee meetings in between for ongoing problem solving.

Traditional Planning	Person-Centered Teams	Circles of Support
Who Initiates the Meeting and for What Purpose?		
Team Leader initiates to meet requirements of regulations.	Organizational change agent initiates to find new directions for the organization.	Focus person, spokesperson, or family member initiates to reach goals they are unable to accomplish working alone.
What Motivates People to Attend the Meeting?		
Avoidance of punishment by regulators. Interest in coordination of departmental units.	Interest in organizational innovation and finding new directions for focus person.	Voluntary commitment by people who are interested in helping someone they care about.
Nature of the Images for the Future:		
Goals will fit within existing program options.	Goals will reflect new program models and options yet to be developed.	Vision will reflect desire of focus person and family.
Roles of Members and Boundaries of Action:		
Members have specific roles and clear boundaries for action. Plans do not change roles or boundaries. Members act within channels of authority already formalized by the organizational structure.	Plans may change roles of members and create new agendas for action. Old boundaries may be changed to allow for new action. Members create new channels and connections to accomplish goals.	Participant roles change constantly based on tasks and circumstances. Boundaries for action are defined by personal vision and commitment of group members. Members use informal networks and contacts to open doors to community.

Traditional Planning	Person-Centered Teams	Circles of Support
Product of an Effective Group Meeting:		
Completed forms and paperwork. Specific goals to use to evaluate program effectiveness.	An agenda for organizational change. A shared understanding of new directions.	Commitments to action by community members. Significant improvement in the life of focus person.
Role of Human Service Worker:		
Set all direction. Organize all activity. Coordinate activities of direct service workers.	Mediate interests of service providers and focus person. Lead organizational change efforts. Listen to direct service workers.	Support directions defined by group. Increase knowledge of available resources. Provide direct services to focus person.
Role of Community Members:		
Not involved in the process.	May help implement some ideas.	Generate and implement plan and action steps.
Role of Person with a Disability or Elder:		
Comply with the plan.	Cooperate in the development of the plan.	Direct plan and activities.

A Circle Building Process

IS	IS NOT
About capacity	About deficiency
A hope for something better with more options and possibilities	An answer to the service system
Empowerment of individuals	Control of individuals
Person-centered	Service-centered
Shared roles within circles	Singular responsibility for activities
Building gifts and connections of people to make things happen	About relying on one overworked manager
A network of people consisting of friends, family, neighbors, and others who know the person best	People who have never seen or been a part of the person's life, but may be connected on paper only
All members are equal, contributing parts of the circle	About titles, power, or position
Interdependent	Dependent
About facilitation: empowering the person, not doing things for the person	About group control
Flexible	Rigid
Bound up in relationships	Bound up in a paper process

A circle of support can provide many wonderful opportunities. One of the most useful discussions revolves around finding ways to increase connections with the local community. In cases where a person is isolated and there is no network from which to draw the circle, this step may have to happen first. If someone already has a number of friends, working to build bridges into community life can still help to broaden a circle and bring in additional opportunities for fun and friendship.

The next section explores the opportunities available in community, and how to access them.

BUILDING BRIDGES

ON FINDING COMMUNITY

Mary E. Hough-Scholl

I didn't set out to find community; all I wanted to do was my laundry. I was new in town and I found a laundromat several blocks from my home. It so happened that next door was a little café that indulged my bad habit. I smoke. It turned out that the people who frequented the café not only smoked but had a passion for Cribbage. I mentioned I play. Someone offered to play. I didn't know it at the time, but I was going to discover two things; one, I didn't play Cribbage as well as I thought; two, I had found community.

Discovering I didn't play well didn't take long. Discovering I was part of a community took a little longer. Looking back I can tell you the foundation was already there the day I walked in. It started with those who opened the café for their own personal reasons. They simply wanted a place they could smoke, get a good cup of coffee, and talk, preferably over a card game. Setting out to create community wasn't on their list of things to do. Like many things in life, it evolved all on its own.

My skill as a Cribbage player improved dramatically, while my inclusion in the core group was so subtle I wasn't even aware it was happening. To tell you the truth, I never really thought of the café in terms of community. That was a concept introduced much later.

So what then was the café? In the beginning for me it was just a place to go. I simply had nothing better to do. I was recovering from a long-term illness so I was only working part time. My children were off going to school. Television just sucked. So for the price of a cup of coffee I could see real people, play cards, and have a conversation. What more could anybody want?

Friends? Friends would be nice. Me, personally, I've always been shy. It's not in my nature to just talk to someone. This does not lend itself to making friends, so the end result was I didn't have any. The great thing about the people at the café was they liked to talk. Me, I listened. This I do well. They also liked to ask questions. Simple ones like How are you doing? What's the weather like? This I could handle. So imagine my surprise when I realized I had gotten to know these people. Some a little bit; some very well. Even more surprising, they had gotten to know me.

How did that happen? It happened because the people who came there didn't have an agenda. They came there just to have a good time. It happened because there was an expectation: that you be yourself. Along with that was the expectation that you must accept others for who they are. This resulted in a large and diverse group.

Of course, with so many personalities conflict is inevitable. Me, I don't do conflict. Luckily others have no problem with it. I sat back and observed and learned. For some it was meet head-on. They would lay all their cards on the table (pun intended). Words would be exchanged. Most not suited for this text. To my surprise, most times that would be it. It seems grudges are not us. Just as often, there were those who would accept that that was just So-and-So being him- or herself and let it go. Almost all brought a sense of humor to the situation. It seemed side-taking was frowned upon. Knowing what was going on in someone's life often helped to keep things in perspective. Allowances would be made when it was known life was difficult in the here-and-now. On the rare occasion the conflict wasn't going to be resolved, both parties would agree to disagree. Mostly anyway. We have lost a few. It seems those who haven't learned to laugh at life, see the other guy's side, or understand they too are human don't stick around.

Unfortunately some do. Community, like family, has those you wish would go away. It's also true that, like family, there are those you have more in common with. Me, I'm a dyed-in-the-wool, true blue UConn Women's Huskies Basketball fan. Something else many of us share. This has given us reason to get together outside the café. For others it's golf or a trip to the casino or, oh-so-many other reasons. The café, however, remains the main meeting place and clearinghouse.

For it is here we bring news that affects our members. The loss of a loved one. An illness. A hospitalization. Cards are put out to be signed. The fund jar set out to help with expenses or for an appropriate gift.

Most importantly, support and understanding are offered. And it is here we celebrate holidays and birthdays, announce the good things in our lives, and occasionally bring our problems.

So we end up commiserating together. Sometimes solutions are offered up, but mostly it's just having someone willing to listen without judgement. Speaking of judgement and, for that matter, diversity, just how tolerant are we? Well, all summer long the Yankee fans bait the Red Sox fans, and both give the Mets fans a hard time. However, it hasn't stopped the Yankee fan from dating the Red Sox fan. Politics is the number one favorite excuse to raise voices and exchange expletives. Open debate is us. The younger generation tends to ignore us old folk but we all know each other's names. Sometimes we even play cards together. Me, I'm so out of the closet, the closet got cobwebs. So far no one has made it an issue. They are, however, curious how I came to have two daughters (tried the straight thing but it didn't take). The non-smokers put up with the smokers. The non-smokers were the minority but the ratio is changing. It seems you can teach an old dog new tricks.

Speaking of changes, we have had a few. Some of the originals have passed away. Some have moved. Some have just moved on. Set Back is as popular as Cribbage these days and the younger crowd prefers Dungeons and Dragons. Me, I work full-time now so I miss many of the day people. Some new faces are showing up. They catch on fast.

All you do is this: pull up a chair, state the game, and introduce yourself. Or, if you are shy like me, just hang around and others will introduce themselves. Or, if you don't know how to play, ask; someone will teach you. Just make sure you bring your sense of humor because it can get bawdy. And just be yourself because you never know where you are going to find community. It may be as close as the nearest café.

Reaching the Island

One objective of the One Candle Power process is to assist someone to enter more completely into the life of the community. Often, the focus of this support is a person with a disability, a family whose child has a disability, or a senior citizen who has lost function due to the aging process. But these principles can be of benefit to anyone, of any age, with or without a disability. For some people, community seems like an island which can be seen but not reached. Therefore, building bridges to community is an important aspect of this work.

One role of a facilitator is to assist each person who cares about the individual to contribute his or her particular gift when the time is right. Some circle members may offer some specific connections to the community. Others may have a different gift. But as opportunities and obstacles are discussed, and strategies are developed, it is important that friends and circle members be encouraged to build bridges into community life wherever possible. A circle facilitator may also be good at linking people with associations and groups, or the facilitator may bring in other people who can act as bridge-builders on the person's behalf.

Here are some simple ways that ordinary folks can use their natural and developed connections to introduce people with disabilities into the associations and neighborhood groups which are found in every community. We hope these examples and hints will stimulate you to be aware of opportunities, and creative in your attempts to bring your family member or friend into full community life.

Using Informal Supports to Involve People in Community

Circle members and friends offer many gifts in the process of building a better future for the focus person. People contribute whatever support they can, and these contributions vary greatly from one situation to another. People can support one another in reaching community by:

- ◆ Bringing their ideas to the group.
- ◆ Bringing their connections to the community, and figuring out creative ways to use these connections.

◆ Helping someone find a job and helping arrange job supports.

◆ Helping individuals and families find respite providers, personal assistants, and other supports.

◆ Helping someone acquire the furniture needed to move into his or her house or apartment.

◆ Helping someone learn to read. Helping with homework.

◆ Helping a person join community associations.

◆ Helping a child become part of the public school system.

◆ Helping a child ride the school bus with the other children.

◆ Programming communication boards with hip words.

◆ Helping someone to move out of a nursing home.

◆ Helping someone start his or her own business.

◆ Helping someone build or join a housing cooperative.

◆ Asking a local reporter to write a story about the person, his or her situation, his or her gifts being offered to the community, and how other people were involved with making this happen.

◆ Representing someone's interest before town meetings and school boards.

◆ Sharing rides to important events.

◆ Helping people interpret policy. Going with the person to interview policymakers about benefit issues, accessibility guidelines, and other issues.

◆ Helping human service agencies become more responsive to people.

◆ Talking on the phone a lot.

◆ Sharing the frustrations people feel as well as celebrating the accomplishments.

◆ Deepening friendships and commitments.

◆ Celebrating birthdays.

From these examples, it is easy to see that more resources become available when members of the group are diverse, representing a variety of connections, perspectives, and ideas. If the group is lacking the right connection, invite someone new to join!

How Do People Make Connections?

All bridge-builders work through a "trust network." Because the members of this network come to trust the bridge-builder, they can help to open doors on behalf of the person with a disability. Building these connections is critical to the long-term goal of increasing community inclusion. These strategies have helped people develop a trust network.

♦ Focus on a neighborhood or some other natural section of the community.

♦ Establish trust networks. Call on people to tell them what you are doing. Ask for ideas and other contacts. Spend a lot of time doing this before making specific requests on behalf of a person.

♦ Join different groups. Pay dues and contribute. Become part of the associational life of the community. Learn about the community and how it works.

♦ Find other "like-minded" groups. Focus on groups that talk about building community. In some cases, religious organizations such as churches may be a good resource.

♦ Find resource manuals and listings of community events. Show up at a lot of events, such as programs sponsored by the local library, civic groups, and associations.

♦ Establish work groups to help think about ideas. Build a circle around a specific individual. Build a community group to help brainstorm. Build a hospitality group to welcome someone into the neighborhood.

♦ Sometimes you can find a grant to work on behalf of a small number of people who want to increase their involvement in the community. This enables local people who are familiar with a particular community to build bridges.

♦ Followup contacts with thank-you notes. Thank people even if nothing comes from the contact right away.

♦ Find ways for people to give of themselves and to give what they know.

What Do Effective Bridge-Builders Have in Common?

♦ Everyone is working through **trust networks** with people who already know each other. People are more likely to open doors for a stranger if that person is recommended by someone they know. If a bridge-builder does not have a network in the geographic or interest area needed by the person, he or she is **taking the time** to build one.

♦ Things work best when the bridge-builder is connected: when he or she is part of the town or organization to which the bridge is being built. **Familiar, trusted people** are in the best position to introduce and escort people with disabilities into new settings and associations. When a bridge-builder is not familiar to existing members, he or she must **find an ally** to help make the connections.

♦ Bridge-builders **take time** to get to know the person they are working to connect. They spend unstructured, personal time with each focus person. The process works best when it is possible to match the interests and choices of the focus person to people and places in the community. Bridge-builders must spend a significant amount of time with the focus person and gain a good understanding of his or her preferences in order to make a good match.

♦ All bridge-builders **start small.** They work with a small number of people at one time so that adequate time and attention can be brought to each individual and situation. Ideally, agencies which support bridge-builders understand the necessity of starting small, and are able to support this approach.

♦ Bridge-building takes **time and patience** before things occur. People must be allowed to work in their own time and in their own way.

♦ Bridge-builders spend most of their **time in the community**. If they work for human service agencies, they have been freed from the demands of the bureaucracy, and are exempt from paperwork and other distractions.

♦ The most effective bridge-builders **are not "professionals**." They are small business owners, hair stylists, local politicians, congregation members, and neighbors. They use common English (not jargon) to describe their feelings and experiences.

♦ **Bridge-builders must be responsive, present, and skilled listeners**. They are opportunity seekers, and they seize every chance to make connections for people. Circles of support provide a unique environment for bridge-building because circle members have already made a **personal commitment** to the individual with a disability. They do their part to make a dream, vision, or goal into a reality by using their existing connections and making new ones.

> Springs are little things, but they are sources of large streams; an acorn is a little thing, but from it can grow a forest of mighty oaks; nails and pegs are little things, but they hold the parts of a large building together; a word, a look, a smile, a frown are all little things, but powerful for good or evil. Think of this, and mind the little things.
>
> - Newell Dwight Hillis

STARTING SMALL

This is what we are about:

We plant seeds that one day will grow.
We water seeds already planted, knowing that they hold future promise.
We lay foundations that will need further development.
We provide yeast that produces effects beyond our capabilities.

We cannot do everything and there is a sense of liberation in realizing that.
This enables us to do something and to do it very well.
It may be incomplete, but it is a beginning, a step along the way,
*   an opportunity for God's grace to enter and do the rest.*

We may never see the end results,
*   but that is the difference between the master builder and the worker.*
We are workers, not master builders, ministers, not messiahs.
We are prophets of a future not our own.

*   -- Monseñor Oscar Romero **

Of all the One Candle Power principles, starting small is the most difficult for us in the West to embrace. We want bigger, better, and more, and we want it now!

All of us who are involved with people with disabilities, whether on a professional or a personal level, want the answers to come quickly. We watch people, particularly those with severe disabilities, wait in frustrating situations because of huge barriers in systems or in communities.

But we have also seen governmental agencies, private groups, or entrepreneurs present THE plan and offer THE way of solving the entire problem at once. These attempts, unfortunately, often end without much

---

*   Text by the late Archbishop Oscar Romero of El Salvador. From a poster distributed by Northern Sun Merchandising, 2916 E. Lake Street, Minneapolis, MN 55406-2065 USA. Used by permission.

result, both for those trying to make the change and for the families and people with disabilities who still continue to wait. We think we must have tangible results or increased profits "by the end of the quarter." When this does not happen, it is considered failure.

In contrast, there is a great deal of wisdom in the Chinese statement of philosophy, "One generation plants the tree in order that the future generation might enjoy the shade."

We in America find this concept difficult to understand and accept. Building for the future in small, solid steps is not a highly regarded approach in our culture. Therefore, we look for big steps, major projects, and heroic answers. These large activities tend to leave ordinary friends, relatives, or neighbors of a person with a disability feeling that they have nothing to offer. They are not going to be able to change the world after all. For that reason, they feel they cannot make much of a difference in the life of a friend or relative with a disability.

We have found this to be just the opposite of what actually happens. Yes, it is important to encourage those among us who are able to change entire systems or make major contributions to use their unique gift. More essential, however, those of us who live on a day-to-day basis with an individual or family need to continue to give our gifts, to share ourselves. Only then, all together, can there be a whole and positive experience for the person with the disability or a family.

There are many examples of the small things people do to overcome a large obstacle. The Berlin Wall did not come down all at once. People may not have had the power to change the way things were, but their heart and spirit were never broken. They worked together in small ways for a long time. Ultimately, the collective voice of people standing in squares, standing up, being counted, fighting for what they believed, overcame the huge obstacle of superior military might and unilateral authority.

This may seem like an extreme example, but little revolutions occur frequently. We believe the small efforts of the people who surround an individual with a disability are far, far more important than that one large and magnificent step which promises to change everything. Again, we are not denying the value of those who wish to make a major contribution. But the effort to find that major contribution should not and must not hinder the gift of ordinary folks in religious communities, neighborhoods, and homes.

The small gifts that we can give are the "lights of hope" that give a person or family the strength to pull through a very difficult path toward full inclusion, respect, and dignity within our society.

There is no magic formula. Instead, there is the work of helping people understand that their gift, however small, is incredibly valuable and very much needed by those with whom they walk and live. Here are some ways to begin:

Start now
Give your gift
Write a note of encouragement
Make a call of friendship
Listen
Give someone a ride
Enjoy each moment together

Start small
Be present
Drop by
Offer a hug
Encourage
Have a good laugh
Walk with someone

No Contribution is Too Small!

Ways to Start Small

Start moving toward the vision NOW. Help members of the group to understand that change takes time and that they will be able to use their capacities to cause change little by little.

Many people may think that being a friend is no big deal. Help them to respect and appreciate the power of simple friendship. Encourage people to give their gifts, while highlighting the importance of just "being there." People may not say much at meetings or have the ability to do anything dramatic. Explain to them that the time to give their gift will come, and that for some people "being present" IS their gift.

Believe in the analogy of nature and its regeneration process: the seed and the small plant are needed in order for the larger plant to develop.

Everybody contributes to the attainment of the dream, even in small or limited ways. This is not a "systems" approach, in which the most efficient plan becomes the goal, and if we do not reach it we have failed. Start where people are and encourage the process to continue. If a person wants to be an astronaut, don't shoot down the dream. Instead, start at the first step and move forward from there.

The process of getting to a dream, vision, or goal is filled with many small victories over many obstacles. The steps are as important as reaching the goal. Pay attention to the small things it takes to work toward a dream.

Celebrate minor accomplishments and encourage people to stay motivated on a difficult path. Small things keep hope alive while creating system change. They also provide stability when circumstances are in flux.

Call often. Send cards often. Be present and responsive as much as possible.

Remember: Small Is Beautiful!

The next two stories illustrate how a vision of the future is reached moment by moment. There is no sudden change in the landscape. Instead, we arrive at our destination quietly and in small increments.

PLOWING THROUGH TO A SOLUTION
Peggy Ludlum

A parent cannot provide everything in a child's or young adult's life. The parent may understand the need for youthful companionship, religious participation with other young people, and the chance for professional success, but he or she cannot just make it happen. These things depend on the caring and efforts of others, and on achievements earned and recognized. Here is where the support of friends comes in. Helping to make dreams come true is hard work, and it takes a lot of effort on the part of other people.

My daughter Cathy wanted to be on her own for a long time, but she seemed to hit a brick wall at every turn. Then she met George Ducharme, Pat Beeman, and Beth Mount and heard about "circles of support." She also learned about personal futures planning, and when she saw her hopes printed out in bright colors on big sheets of paper, she immediately began to feel that she had more going for her than she had thought. It took five years of meetings; intensive planning; help from Sarah Page, Co-op Initiatives, and the Developmental Disabilities Council; and the energy of devoted friends to make Cathy's dream of independence possible.

Along the way, we both had many experiences and learned many things. Cathy and her circle members were invited to speak in Maryland and Montreal, and off she went in our old van. There was much planning involved around her personal care needs on these trips. I trusted that her friends would be there for her. Mainly, I was worried about the van breaking down, but everything went fine. Then they were invited to Ohio, which was too far to drive, and off they went in an airplane.

Gradually, Cathy began hiring her own personal assistants. She took another step toward independence by opening her own consulting business. These experiences and the encouragement of so many people gave her the confidence to make the big move into the housing co-op and change her life.

Three years ago, I had to be hospitalized suddenly for several days, and Cathy's circle was wonderful in pitching in and helping out. Her circle of support has been my support as well.

This has meant a great deal to me as I am getting older. Cathy needs a good deal of help which I am really no longer able to provide. Many of the people in her circle have young children, jobs, and homes to take care of. I don't know how they are able to accomplish all this and still make the time for us. I am forever grateful for their contagious and tireless optimism, refusal to accept discouragement or defeat, and ability to just keep on plowing through to a solution.

---

* This article was drawn from a talk my mother gave at the "Third Half of Life" conference in 1992. Though she was always a very important and supportive part of my circle, she preferred to stay out of the spotlight. It was a blessing to find the notes she had prepared for this presentation.

KANSAS STORIES
Lorene Castle

After hearing several Connecticut stories about circles of support, I realized that they reminded me of living in a farm community in Kansas.

I went to high school with 13 other classmates, two of whom were twins. One of the twins was in an automobile accident a few years after he graduated. I remember visiting his family at the hospital shortly before my son was born 27 years ago. Tony had a head injury, and in those days the emergency team could not get him to a hospital with the speed that is common today. Tony was in a coma from which he never woke up. The doctors told the family that they should put Tony in a nursing home because no brain activity was detected.

But Tony's family had a dream. They wanted to have Tony live at home for as long as God intended Tony could live. Three years ago, when I went home to visit, my mother asked her friends over for a picnic. Rosemary couldn't come because she was staying with Tony so his mother could go to a meeting at church. Lola told me this spring that Tony's mother would not go to the basement during the recent tornadoes that hit Kansas because she wouldn't leave Tony.

I share this story because this is a dream that most of us would say is too difficult to pursue; but one family, with the help of friends and relatives, has made their dream a reality for over 27 years.

Another Kansas story involves my mother and her friends, who all share a dream of living in their own homes for as long as they live. My mother's friends are all 70 to 85 years old. They live alone on their farms, and their nearest neighbors are usually one to two miles away. They have the usual physical problems of people in this age group, so they call each other daily. My mother's phone was often busy when I called, and this irritated me until I realized that these women had created a circle of support for each other.

They decide among themselves who will accompany whom to the doctor's office. One member of the circle told me confidentially that my mother was no longer a safe driver. I suggested that she offer to drive my mother's car. Now, when it's my mother's turn to drive, her car is driven by Rosemary.

The circle changes over time, but remains intact. One member died from cancer. When I visited the next year, I met a new woman who had joined the "circle."

One member had a lot of money, and another had lost most of her money due to the Kansas farm economy in the 1980s. The members of the circle used their senior citizen discounts and coupons so they could all go to dinner. No one felt excluded because of unavailability of financial resources.

So far only one member of the circle lives in a nursing home. I saw her this summer, and she was able to fill me in on how the other women were doing.

And so it goes in Kansas as well as Connecticut.

This story was taken from the Communitas Communicator, Fall 1991.

CHANGING SYSTEMS

Most of the strategies described until this point can be useful for everyone in every situation. Providing **leadership**, looking at people's **capacities**, planning a **future,** starting a **circle of support, building bridges** to community opportunities, and **starting small** are consistently beneficial, no matter where we live, no matter who we are, and whether we have a disability or not.

The seventh strategy, **changing systems**, may also be necessary for a person or family to accomplish the identified vision. This is not always the case. We have found, however, that for many people, laws, policies, regulations, or agency practices may stand in the way of achieving a particular dream for the future. When this happens, there is a need to help people with similar issues to join forces and work toward removing these barriers.

This process is extremely difficult, and calls upon everyone in a circle of support to stand together and walk the long, arduous road to a satisfactory conclusion. We have walked with many people whose stories include creative solutions to a system obstacle. Several detailed stories appear on the following pages, but a summary of several additional stories may help to set the stage.

> A life spent making mistakes is not only more honorable but more useful than a life spent doing nothing.
>
> George Bernard Shaw

♦ Mary-Ann and Raymond both had major problems caused by policies of the State vocational rehabilitation agency. Together with their circles of support, they were able to negotiate creative new funding options which are now being used to help others with severe physical disabilities to find and maintain employment.

♦ Regina, a young woman who was living in a nursing home, was one of a number of people who expressed the wish to live in the community. The primary barrier for them was that State programs providing personal assistance services offered only a very limited number of hours. Everyone in this group needed more hours than could be paid for under this policy. There were no easy solutions. But heroic advocacy efforts by a number of circles of support and grassroots advocacy groups led to a pilot project which helped Regina and several other people leave institutions and return to the community. By combining informal community supports, technology to allow control of the home environment, and paid support hours, Regina and many others have been able to live richer, fuller lives.

The energy and time needed to change laws, regulations, and policies literally drive people together to support one another, each doing his or her small part. Just as circles of support help individuals work cooperatively on behalf of their friend, people facing similar systems obstacles need to help one another to change that system. By banding together and working with other advocacy organizations, they can begin doing what is necessary to begin the long, slow process of changing an agency's policy or direction.

In Connecticut, people with disabilities have presented their own stories and issues to key decisionmakers by

◆ Attending state- and federally-initiated forums on housing, work options, inclusive education, and general policy issues

◆ Developing their own forums and inviting legislators and policy people from the appropriate agencies

◆ Participating in legislative coffees, meeting individually with legislators, and constantly writing letters and making phone calls about the need to redirect funding so that people can receive personal assistance services in the community

◆ Providing individual viewpoints about the impact of pending laws and regulations on specific people with disabilities

It is crucial that people with disabilities, their families, friends, neighbors, and members of their circles of support feel that they have the potential to change federal, state, and local laws, regulations, and bureaucracies. While the process is never easy, feeling powerless will not get people anywhere. And those in policymaking roles are also human beings, and when presented with an individual story, complete with all of its struggles, they cannot help but be affected. They may not be able to make the change we want without approval of the legislature, the Governor, etc., but it never hurts to get people on our side. Then it is off to convince the legislature and the Governor!

The path to a specific dream of inclusion in community life consists of <u>both</u> seeking systems change <u>and</u> trying creative options generated by a circle of friends.

With the help of his circle of support, Raymond "Todd" Kilroy presented testimony to the U.S. Senate on April 8, 1987. If one reads Public Law 100-146, the <u>Developmental Disabilities Assistance and Bill of Rights Act Amendments of 1987</u>, the impact of his statement below can be more fully understood.

> "I ask you to re-authorize the Developmental Disabilities Act and to expand its ability to empower individuals and families to control our own futures. I ask you to move the developmental disabilities program away from providing service toward empowering me and families to acquire the support we want. I ask you to move the developmental disabilities program away from enhancing specialized disability organization to adapting generic neighborhood associations."

Upon reading the full text of Raymond's testimony, John McKnight of Northeastern University wrote on May 22, 1987, "It is the most significant statement of our goals that I have ever seen. Would you tell Raymond how much I am impressed by his statement. I will be copying it and sending it to people throughout the United States."

CONFRONTING SYSTEM BARRIERS

What happens when we confront a system-based barrier that seems "too big" for the group, "too complex" for anyone to understand, or just "too frustrating" for people to tackle? There are no secret formulas for dissolving these barriers. The only answer is more hard work.

Here are some strategies that often help when we face complex systems issues.

1. **ORGANIZE A FORUM** – This is a way to bring policy people and other stakeholders together to discuss obstacles and opportunities affecting a number of people in many different circles. Forums can be held about housing issues, integration of public schools, community building, or any other topic where policies may need changing. Forums focus the issue by bringing those with differing perspectives together, and creating a common understanding of the problems people with disabilities and their families face.

> Finding capacity is not the same as ignoring difficulty. Change requires action to affect the world as it is, not as one would like it to be.
>
> Yes, I Can Booklet,
> Community Regeneration Project,
> Rodale Institute, PA

2. **HAVE A MEETING AND BRING A FRIEND** – A number of people working on the same issue can set up meetings with key decisionmakers who have influence over the use of funding. People with disabilities go to meet with these folks and often take one or two friends with them. They ask questions of the key people, raise issues, and generally make themselves known. Find ways to call a meeting with the policy people and outline the issues faced by you, your family member, or your friend. Try to get commitments. Plan a followup activity (a thank-you letter, sending additional information, planning another meeting, etc.) so your visit is not forgotten.

3. **CREATE A TASK FORCE** – Don't wait for someone else to take the lead. Find other people who share the same frustrations. Join together and strategize. Network! Then put your enthusiasm into action.

4. MAKE SOME POLICY RECOMMENDATIONS

– Submit a policy analysis statement to an appropriate governmental body, or a member of the state or federal legislature. This statement should provide a summary of the systems issues emerging from individuals and groups working on similar barriers. Include a number of recommendations for future policy development. Be sure that your issues are represented in these reports.

5. KEEP MEETING

– In the face of seemingly immovable obstacles, it is good to have a circle of support or similar network to keep hopes alive. Working on systems barriers is often so frustrating that people may want to give up. Keep meeting. Keep brainstorming. Look for another angle to the issue. Talk to other people about it and get some new blood involved.

6. INVITE KEY PEOPLE TO MEET WITH YOU ON YOUR TURF

– Get together with your friends or circle members and invite the people with the power to meet with you. Hold the meeting in your living room, or depending on the circumstances, in your parents' living room, a local church or library, or even the nursing home conference room. Get the policymakers into the picture and tell them what is really going on. Let them know how important these issues are to you and your friends. Ask them to brainstorm with you.

7. LOOK FOR COMMUNITY-BUILDING ALTERNATIVES

– Sometimes a systems issue takes so long to resolve that we find solutions in the local community which meet our needs just as well, if not better. Look for these opportunities. Think about community solutions first, then look to the system for answers as a last resort.

8. CONTINUE TO DISCOVER WHAT WORKS AND

> Realize that change is not always a process of improvement.
> Sometimes it is a process of invention.
> When Thomas Edison invented the light bulb, he didn't start by trying to improve the candle.
> He decided that he wanted better light and went from there.
>
> Wendy Kopp,
> Founder of Teach for America

SHARE IT – Continue learning effective ways to influence the system. Network meetings will provide a way for people to share victories as well as frustrations. Continue to document effective strategies.

9. BUILD A WEB PAGE – Share your ideas and resources, both locally and nationally. Find other people interested in the same issues. Increase information and opportunities for change.

> Tell me and I will forget;
> Show me and I may remember;
> Involve me and I will know.
>
> Chinese proverb

COMMUNITY-CENTERED CHANGE

Systems change, as we have defined it over the last fifteen years, is aimed at urging government and private agencies to provide more opportunities for people with disabilities to be included in ordinary community life, sharing the freedom guaranteed to all of us in great works such as the U.S. Constitution.

The following quote from Mary O'Connell's book *The Gift of Hospitality* clearly distinguishes between "organized service systems" and "the free space of human relationships called community."

> In a social service system, people are known by what's wrong: by their condition or label. **In community**, people are known as individuals.

> In a system, people are incomplete and need to be changed or "fixed." **In community**, people are as they are, with opportunities to follow their own dreams.

> In a system, relationships are unequal; service workers do things "for" clients and don't look for any contribution in return. **In community**, relationships are reciprocal, give and take; and the diverse gifts of many people are recognized.

> In a system, people are broken into parts and separated into groups. **In community**, people have the chance to be accepted as whole persons and viewed as part of the whole society.

> In a system, problems are solved by consulting authorities, policies, procedures. **In community**, people seek answers from their own experience and the wisdom of others.

In a system, there is no room to acknowledge mistakes and uncertainty; information is communicated in professional jargon that distances individuals from their actions. **In community**, people can make honest efforts and acknowledge honest mistakes and fears.

In a system, all problems have a rational solution. **In community**, there is room for confusion and mystery, and a recognition that some things are beyond human control.

Community, finally, is no different for people with disabilities than for any of the rest of us. It is the free space where people think for themselves, dream their dreams and come together to create and celebrate their common humanity.

The next story describes the 13-year process of creating a new living option for people with severe disabilities in Connecticut. It shows the long periods of waiting, the frustrations, and the compromises which are sometimes necessary when trying to change a service system.

LONG JOURNEY HOME
Cathy Ludlum

I can't believe it.

I wander around the courtyard, which is still strewn with bricks, bits of plywood and metal, and other construction debris. The ground is unplanted and sandy, and I have to watch where I'm going or risk getting gloriously stuck in what will be my own front yard.

I make my way around the huge dumpster to look at the four buildings. Two stories high, they are beige brick on the first floor and stucco above. Some windows are open to let out the smell of drying paint. The front doors are white; about half of them are on now, and cabinets are being installed.

I tour what will be my unit. My desk will go here, my bed there. I look out onto the porch and picture the yellow tomatoes I want to grow next summer.

I can touch the walls, but I still can't believe it.

Sometime in the next two months I will be moving into my own home, into a housing cooperative.

Thirteen years ago, I was a high school student thinking about getting out on my own. I was wondering what would happen to me after my mother could no longer assist me with daily activities such as bathing and dressing.

Ten years ago I was busy with college, but in my spare time I researched housing options in preparation for my big move. I wrote to specialized complexes thousands of miles away, consulted with counselors and occupational therapists. Everyone told me what I already knew: that with my limited dexterity and significant breathing problems there was no way I could live without an extraordinary amount of support. I took this to mean paid support. I worked out budgets for 24-hour assistance, but they were so distressing that I threw them away.

Seven years ago I graduated from college. It should have been a joyous time, but it felt like the end of everything. After six years of housing research, I had not found any situation which would meet both my need for safety and my need to retain control over my life. So I finally gave up the search, and with it any hope I had for continued life in the community.

When my mom could no longer care for me I would go to a nursing home. It wasn't what I wanted, but it seemed inevitable.

Then, five years ago, I went to a conference where I heard David Wetherow speak on housing cooperatives. He talked about mutual support, about how people with disabilities could not only receive, but also give support to their non-disabled neighbors. He talked about home ownership (something I had never even considered), and about autonomy, security, and community. I listened, afraid to hope, but afraid not to.

It was also at this conference that the idea of "circles of support" came to Connecticut. At the end of the conference, I wrote on the evaluation form that I would like to know more about co-ops. Two months later, Pat Beeman, George Ducharme, and Beth Mount were in my living room, asking me to describe my vision of the future. I wanted to live in a housing co-op, have adequate personal assistance, and work at a job where I could reach my full potential. They said these were great dreams, and asked me to invite some of my friends to walk along with us.

And that was when things started to happen. The first order of business was to find out "What exactly is a housing co-op and are there any in Connecticut?" We all set out to find the answers, but there was something different about the search now. We were all embarking on it together. As we went along, we shared the progress we made as well as the obstacles we encountered. We talked on the phone; we carpooled to meetings; we wrote notes; we had parties. When one of us got discouraged, there were others to talk to and draw strength from.

After awhile George connected us with Sarah Page, a consultant who specialized in housing co-ops. She, in turn, discovered that although Connecticut had many co-ops, none was accessible to people who use wheelchairs. She networked with many local non-profit groups to see if they might be willing to develop an accessible co-op which I could apply to, but all roads ended in dead ends.

With my circle's encouragement, Sarah pulled together a board of directors and created a non-profit organization, Co-op Initiatives, Inc. The first project of this group was to develop a co-op which emphasized accessibility and mutual support. Unfortunately, given state and federal law, it could have been a serious conflict of interest for me or other members of my circle who wanted to apply to the co-op to serve on the non-profit board. Realizing that our participation could jeopardize our standing as applicants, as well as the legal position of Co-op Initiatives, we gave up our active role. We advised on the design of the co-op, especially as it related to accessibility, and watched the progress eagerly, but were not as involved as we would otherwise have been.

Meanwhile, my circle and I were receiving invitations to travel and speak about what was happening in our lives as a result of this process. As circle members drove my van and assisted me with personal tasks, I discovered that my needs were not as complex as I had always thought. As long as I was with people who were willing to listen to me, I would be fine. Gradually, I came to believe that with a combination of paid assistants and less formal help from friends, I could make it in the community after all.

With the backing of my circle, I started hiring my own personal assistants, a step I had always considered too risky to think about. The change in my lifestyle was remarkable. I was able to travel across Connecticut without my mother; to wash my hair and change my clothes without consulting her schedule; to go shopping, to the park, or wherever I wanted to go.

And the people in my circle, always concentrating on my capacities instead of my deficiencies, started giving me writing and editing assignments, and offering to pay me! At first I refused, afraid to lose Medicare benefits, but after a year or so I found myself thinking about starting my own business. I got a Macintosh computer and expanded my services to include layout work for newsletters, brochures, and flyers.

After a long and frustrating site search, Co-op Initiatives bought the perfect piece of land in Manchester. It is flat and wooded, in a quiet residential neighborhood, yet only one block from Main Street. Plans were drawn up, showing four 4-unit buildings, with four accessible units scattered throughout the complex. It was starting to get exciting!

Now the lengthy application process began. Last November I attended a public meeting about the project. I was a nervous wreck for days as I filled out the application form because there was no guarantee that I would be accepted into the co-op. The application is similar to a mortgage application, requiring detailed information about credit history, present landlord, and employment status, as well as short essays about community spirit. I wanted mine to be worded perfectly.

After several tense weeks, I was called for my first interview. Snow was falling as I crunched around looking for the accessible door to the church. I don't remember the interview except that there were six of them and only one of me, and that they asked what I would do if a pipe burst in my unit. This got to be a joke later because so many of us, including me, said we would call a plumber. The correct answer is, of course, to *shut off the water valve!*

The second interview was much less frightening. Two members of the selection committee came over to inspect my present residence and chat briefly about my expectations of co-op life.

Finally, the call came asking me to participate with some other applicants in a role play exercise. We all passed, and were accepted as co-op candidates, although we will not officially be "members" until we have completed all our sweat equity requirements. In our development, that means 200 hours of work in addition to a $500 down-payment.

The summer and fall have been crammed full of sweat equity activities. Every Thursday night the candidates meet for a two-hour training. The trainings are intended to prepare us to own and manage our co-op, and cover such topics as running meetings, effective communication and decision making, and house rules. These trainings will continue until March.

On weekends we have been doing sweat equity at the construction site. In 100-degree July heat, August rain, and September chill, we turned out to help build one another's homes. We swept up and tossed debris into the dumpster, installed insulation, and gave all the units one coat of paint. For everyone, it meant an investment of time and energy. For me, it also meant recruiting and organizing volunteers to do sweat equity on my behalf. But I loved being at the site, and went almost every week.

Sweat equity involves working on the building, but it is also a way of getting to know your neighbors. Through countless hours of shared experience, bonds are created which will hold the co-op together over time. And this is why I wanted to live in a co-op in the first place.

We're coming down to the end now. Except for the landscaping, our work at the site is about over. It will be up to the contractors to finish the skilled labor and put on the final touches. Our projected moving date is January 1.

Through an outrageous set of circumstances that would take an hour to explain, I've found an assistant to live with me. She is young and enthusiastic, and we already have a very congenial working relationship. People I know have given me some furniture and other household items to help me get started, and I am not lacking anything I really need. Finances are a worry, but then again, everyone I know is also struggling to make ends meet.

So the only thing left is to actually move! There is this feeling of anticlimax as I wait for the last few pieces to fall into place. For thirteen years I've been hoping to have my own home, and now I'm weeks away. I'm looking forward to moving day, and to shared meals in the community room with my neighbors. I have always wanted to prepare big holiday dinners and invite a lot of people from one- and two- person families. It won't be long now 'till I can.

And once I'm settled, and coping with all these new things (like cooking and laundry), I will start working on a whole new set of dreams!

This story originally appeared in the *Communitas Communicator*, Vol. 2, No. 3, Fall 1991.

ROOM TO GROW

Cathy Ludlum

I wandered from table to table in the crowded classroom, looking and listening intently, trying to take everything in.

There was a futuristic model house, a comparative study of China and Japan, and a detailed family tree.

A girl pointed to Morse Code dots on a large piece of colored cardboard, and demonstrated a working telegraph she had made.

Another girl, sitting beside a large aquarium that contained two hermit crabs, discussed her interest in marine biology. She showed me her report comparing the behavior of the land-dwelling hermit crab with that of its underwater cousin.

One boy had studied the architecture of castles; another displayed a series of reports on classical composers.

A girl had portrayed an owl (the school mascot) in cross-stitch.

There were portfolios of paintings, books of poetry, videotapes of dance.

This was the exhibition put on each year by the 4th, 5th, and 6th graders in my town's "gifted" classes. The projects were wonderful and imaginative, the students proud, the audience attentive, yet something about the whole thing bothered me.

I have known for a while now that all students belong together, that children should not be separated by perceived ability or disability, and that was part of why I felt uncomfortable.

But there was something else. It was more subtle … and I spent most of the summer trying to figure out what it was.

Then a friend, without realizing it, made the issue clear to me in two sentences. "I don't want to be treated 'special,'" he said. "I want to be treated like everyone else."

He was telling me how hard he had to work to fit in at a job that he was not really suited for. And I was thinking about what a talented person he is, and wondering why it seemed impossible for him to make a living doing things which were compatible with his personality, talents, and dreams.

Then it hit me.

Our schools, workplaces, and other social structures are organized to treat everyone the same. As a result, anyone who is different - has a disability label, or a gifted label, or both, or a label of another kind – is treated as special and therefore stands out.

But that's backwards!
Everybody is special!
Why not turn it around?

Why not abandon the cookie-cutter approach to education, work, housing, support services, transportation, and recreation? You don't have to look far to see that uniformity doesn't work.

Why not give every student the opportunity to do a year-long project about art, history, science, or anything else he or she may be interested in?

Why not create a workplace where every person's gifts are nurtured, where talkative people can talk, quiet people can be quiet, creative people can be creative, and everyone is accepted and valued?

Why not develop neighborhoods where people's gifts are recognized and multiplied, where relationships grow, and everyone fits in?

Why not make sure all services are provided in the homes, work environments, and leisure settings people have chosen for themselves?

Why not???

This story originally appeared in the *Communitas Communicator*, Vol. 2, No. 3, Fall 1991.

PERSONAL SUPPORT: NOTHING CAN HAPPEN WITHOUT PEOPLE

A vision by itself is just a pretty idea on paper. Nothing can happen without encouragement, listening, and talking it through. It is important that people have others around them who can stay awhile, pursue the vision with them, and help them through the feelings that accompany any transition. We may know we want the vision, but especially for people with disabilities, there are so many more factors that confront us along with the positive changes.

It will take MUCH SUPPORT AND ENCOURAGEMENT to build that vision and cross that bridge to a better place. A commitment to people is about something more than professional labels, status, and even pay. If we say, "This is somebody else's job to make this happen. Why am I devoting time to it?" then there isn't a sense of commitment and caring in our relationship with that individual. Commitment means putting ourselves at the side of that person; his or her struggle becomes our struggle also.

It is important to be a friend because we like the person, not because he or she needs our kindness. If I were with you because I liked you, but you were only willing to be with me because you felt sorry for me, we could not be friends. You are not my friend because you do me favors. Instead, you want to do me favors because you are my friend.

Responsiveness to people's situations does not limit itself to 8:30-4:30, or whatever hours we normally work. The challenges and feelings one goes through during a transition may happen at any time. Sometimes there isn't a specific thing you can do while going through a rough spot, but maybe all that is needed is support and presence from someone who cares. Sometimes it is a waiting game.

We need to listen to what the other person says to us, but sometimes we listen best when no words are spoken.

> If we take people
> as we find them,
> we make them worse,
> but
> if we treat them
> as though they are
> what they should be,
> we help them to become
> what they are
> capable of becoming.
>
> Goethe

We listen for that silent message of feeling. We listen for pain expressed in sighs or other gestures not associated with joy. We listen for desires which may be expressed in the language of the eyes.

Above all, people are people. Some of us have disabilities and others do not. But we all go through the same things when change is happening in our lives. We have ambivalent feelings, and need reassurance that everything is okay.

WHAT HAS ONE CANDLE POWER ACCOMPLISHED OVER TIME?

In the beginning, this was all just theory. Ideas were put into practice in the lives of people, but none of us really knew whether bringing people together, expressing a vision, connecting with community, and taking small steps toward a dream would make a difference in people's lives.

Nothing works all the time for everyone, and One Candle Power is no exception. We will explore the difficulties in Part III of this book. But the use of these principles has changed the way we as people with disabilities see ourselves, and how we are seen by others. As people have gathered in small groups in homes, libraries, churches, and synagogues, many important things have happened within agencies, organizations, and communities. The dreams of children and adults with disabilities are being brought closer to reality.

Here are some examples:

♦ A statewide pilot project to allow people to hire their own personal assistants was started. Gradually, this concept has taken hold so that more people now have the choice of hiring and supervising their own support people.

♦ A non-profit agency was created to

> Far better it is to dare mighty things, to win glorious triumphs, even though checkered by failure, than take rank with those poor spirits who neither enjoy much nor suffer much, because they live in the gray twilight that knows not victory nor defeat.
>
> Theodore Roosevelt

develop accessible, affordable, integrated housing cooperatives. In 2002, this agency has completed four co-ops and a fifth is underway. Many other housing options, such as Home of Your Own, have given people with disabilities more choices about where to live.

♦ Respite needs of some families have been met through informal meetings and celebrations which brought together members of many circles of support.

♦ A state vocational rehabilitation agency has become more aware and sensitive to the needs of people with severe disabilities.

♦ Increased education and sensitivity of state and local housing officials to the needs of people with disabilities as individuals, not just as a group

♦ Involvement of church groups and other faith networks, supporting families so that caregivers can go away on vacation

♦ A chance to live outside of the institution, bringing dignity, respect, and freedom to individuals

♦ Inclusion of children in neighborhood schools and regular education classes

♦ Development of creative housing options such as mixed-income housing cooperatives (they said it couldn't be done!), or leasing of the family home to a son or daughter with necessary supports

♦ Community education brought about by involvement in meetings of circles of support

♦ Exploration of creative ways to resolve insurance problems, explore employment options, and solve personal assistance issues

♦ Productive and meaningful employment for people with severe disabilities within non-profit organizations, state agencies, and community businesses; employment which allows people to use their many abilities: not "busy-work"

♦ Networking with local officials, neighborhood members, and other local groups about an individual's desires and how to make them come true

♦ Development of more natural friendships and supports

During our fifteen years of walking with people, there have been many times that we have experienced a phenomenon which can best be described as the blowing out of our candle. A strong wind comes along in the form of exhaustion, discouragement, frustration, lost opportunities, or other problems, and we find ourselves sitting in the dark, ready to give up. This is when the strength and capacities of our fellow travellers come to bear. We have found that there is always someone ready to share his or her candle with another, to ignite the smoldering wick once again. Our strength is renewed, and together we embark on the next part of the journey.

Have patience with everything unresolved in your heart
and try to love the questions themselves ...
Don't search for the answers,
which could not be given to you now,
because you would not be able to live them.
And the point is, to live everything.
Live the questions now.
Perhaps then, someday far in the future,
you will gradually, without even noticing it,
live your way into the answer.

Rainer Maria Rilke

PART II:

IMPERFECT CHANGE

WELCOME TO HOLLAND

I am often asked to describe the experience of raising a child with a disability - to try to help people who have not shared that unique experience to understand it, to imagine how it would feel. It's like this......

When you're going to have a baby, it's like planning a fabulous vacation trip - to Italy. You buy a bunch of guide books and make your wonderful plans. The Coliseum. The Michelangelo David. The gondolas in Venice. You may learn some handy phrases in Italian. It's all very exciting.

After months of eager anticipation, the day finally arrives. You pack your bags and off you go. Several hours later, the plane lands. The stewardess comes in and says, "Welcome to Holland."

"Holland?!?" you say. "What do you mean Holland?? I signed up for Italy! I'm supposed to be in Italy. All my life I've dreamed of going to Italy."

But there's been a change in the flight plan. They've landed in Holland and there you must stay.

The important thing is that they haven't taken you to a horrible, disgusting, filthy place, full of pestilence, famine and disease. It's just a different place.

So you must go out and buy new guide books. And you must learn a whole new language. And you will meet a whole new group of people you would never have met.

It's just a different place. It's slower-paced than Italy, less flashy than Italy. But after you've been there for a while and you catch your breath, you look around.... and you begin to notice that Holland has windmills....and Holland has tulips. Holland even has Rembrandts.

But everyone you know is busy coming and going from Italy... and they're all bragging about what a wonderful time they had there. And for the rest of your life, you will say "Yes, that's where I was supposed to go. That's what I had planned."

And the pain of that will never, ever, ever, ever go away... because the loss of that dream is a very very significant loss.

But... if you spend your life mourning the fact that you didn't get to Italy, you may never be free to enjoy the very special, the very lovely things ... about Holland.

DREAMS, DISILLUSIONMENT, AND GROWTH

The story on the previous page is often used to describe the shock people go through when they have a first-hand experience with disability, either their own or that of a loved one. But the analogy can be carried farther. We think we know how things "should be," and when something is not that way, it is jarring to us.

One Candle Power has made it acceptable for individuals and families to dream of a better life. The vision is drawn out, the course is set, and off we go in pursuit of something truly beautiful. The path is difficult, but we are strengthened by the knowledge that when we finally get there – to our own home, our happier job, our involvement with the Historical Society – it will be a wondrous and amazing thing.

And it is... to a point.

Surmounting obstacles to attain a vision is always a victory; but it is never a total victory. The reality of life, whether you have a disability or not, is that what you envision and what you get cannot be the same. There are misunderstandings, arguments, disappointments in abundance. Does that mean the dream was not worth the effort?

Most people would say no, that having goals to reach toward is an essential part of life. Without hope, despair would prevail; without action, nothing would change. Most would say that the journey in itself brought lessons and joys of great value, and attaining a dream and finding it imperfect is better than not daring to try.

Beth Mount and friends wrote about this phenomena in 1990, and many others have expanded on this theme. In this section, you will find the other half of the stories begun in Part I:

Arriving at the threshold of a dream…
Entering in…
Enjoying the good…
Shouldering new responsibilities…
Bearing them well…
Bearing them badly…
Wishing for more…

Living with Tensions

Working for personal and social change is usually a big mess. The journey involves a balance between having hope and the pursuit of a dream, while living with the limitations of reality, such as poverty, discrimination, and personal rejection. In addition, it often takes years to make powerful personal and systemic change, and the amount of waiting can wear people down. Person-centered work brings us closer to the people we intend to support and challenges us to feel what they feel. As we learn to "walk with" people rather than "rule over" them, we may be exposed to tensions and feelings that are difficult for us.

In seeking to respond to people rather than services, we often find ourselves aching from the tensions between our ideals and the realities we face. This pain tends to push us toward two extremes: we may become distracted by sentimental daydreams about what is happening, or feel trapped by despair over the realities people face. Either extreme leaves us paralyzed. The energy for change requires balancing these opposites: hope and despair, vision and reality, the future and the present, celebration and mourning.

Personal stories of change seem filled with imperfection. Things don't go as we planned. If we are lucky, we have as many positive surprises as we have disappointments, and we make progress in spite of limitations. If we are not so lucky, the disappointments outnumber the gains. We sit month after month, year after year, in the same place. Perhaps we hold onto our hope, but we feel sad and helpless. We take the time to celebrate and search for reasons to laugh. We must not jump ship because we cannot face our sense of helplessness. Things *do* change when we sustain our commitment.

The Tensions of Person-Centered Change
Beth Mount

IDEAL/IMPERATIVE	REALITY/CHALLENGE
EMBRACING CONFUSION when people try to live decent lives in a society that devalues the contributions of its older citizens and members who are labeled with disabilities	**WALKING WITH PEOPLE** through the struggle, loneliness, and rejection that comes from taking a stand, such as reclaiming one's personhood
FINDING CAPACITIES IN EVERY PERSON, seeing the contribution each person has to make in community life, no matter who they are and how many limitations they face	**BEING DISILLUSIONED** by how ill-equipped systems are to support people in living a life that expresses their gifts and desires; SEEING THROUGH any promise of a quick fix for the injustice people face.
INSPIRING HOPE BY FINDING A PERSONAL VISION FOR THE FUTURE that can sustain people to work together over time to build a better future for themselves and their communities	**FACING DISAPPOINTMENT** when finding how little support most people really have to pursue a dream
FINDING RICHNESS in DAY-TO-DAY LIFE, starting small by finding the things we can change and encouraging responsiveness in relationships	**CONFRONTING BIG BARRIERS** by challenging the community and societal structures that limit people
MAKING TIME FOR MUSIC, ART, CREATIVITY, HUMOR, AND LAUGHTER and many ways to bring beauty and pleasure into the process of change	**DISTURBING THINGS** and facing the discomfort that comes with breaking the rules
CREATING OCCASIONS FOR CELEBRATION AND HOSPITALITY to sustain us on the journey	**STRENGTHENING RESISTANCE** by getting clear about those things we will not do

Many things have changed for the Meadows Family since Kevin's inclusion in a regular high school was featured in the first *One Candle Power* series. As sometimes happens, a period of great victory and involvement in the community was followed by a time of significant struggle. Below, Linda shares how the family is coping in light of new circumstances.

LIVING IN THE HOLE
Linda Meadows

After Kevin got out of high school, things went really well for a couple of years. As often happens, little gestures by caring people made a difference. Through a friend, Kevin got a job delivering interoffice mail at the local community college. In order for him to deliver the mail effectively, he needed a tray with different compartments to attach to his wheelchair. One of Kevin's old high school teachers approached a woodworking student about making the tray. My husband, Carl, and I developed a cardboard prototype, and the student made the tray.

Part of what worked about the college job was that Kevin was able to select his own support person to accompany him at work. We were going through a small agency that provided job coaches, but where the individuals receiving support had a lot of control over what happened. Funding was provided through our state vocational rehabilitation agency from a small program designed to help people who would otherwise fall through the cracks.

What did not work was that I had to drive Kevin to the college every morning and pick him up in the afternoon. We live way out, so this was a bit of a hike each time. Our van was old, having about 110,000 miles on it already; and we were stretching it out as long as we could because we didn't know how we would be able to afford a new one. After a year or two, we became concerned that driving such a distance every day was eventually going to leave us with no transportation at all. Although we were delighted with our little support agency, we needed to change to a larger agency which offered lift-equipped van pickup as part of its employment support service.

Unfortunately, changing to the new agency meant that Kevin no longer had a say in who accompanied him to work. He was assigned people who were not able to give him the physical support he needed. Worse, his support people did not appear to think of him as a full human being, with his own ideas, preferences, and dreams. Things started to go downhill, and Kevin's job at the college eventually ended.

The support agency transferred Kevin to a sheltered workshop, where he spent all day with many other people with severe disabilities and a couple of staff people. After Kevin's great inclusion experience in high school, and a couple of years working at the college, it was a blow to return to the world of disability segregation. We asked the agency to look into small businesses in the area where Kevin might be able to offer his services, but there was no followup.

So Kevin worked in a thrift store, sorting through dirty old shoes. Due to the nature of the work, all the employees were required to wear gloves, but somehow Kevin would never get any. Adding insult to injury, the staff person who assisted Kevin to eat at lunchtime insisted on wearing rubber gloves. This was both humiliating and physically uncomfortable, and Kevin would gag whenever the rubber came near to his face. After endless complaining from us, someone else was finally assigned to assist him with lunch.

We struggled for years to find a way for Kevin to have a job in the community once again. Transportation has always been an issue because we live a distance from the nearest city. There are no buses, so there is no dial-a-ride service either. If a family is not able to afford an adapted vehicle, the person with a disability just sits home. We have recently been able to replace our old van with a more reliable vehicle, but this doesn't solve everything because I am still needed to drive Kevin everywhere.

Employment support for community settings (not sheltered workshops) is extremely difficult to come by. Since Kevin did not have a label of mental retardation, he did not qualify for much in the way of job coaching or other work supports. Most people with disabilities other than mental retardation use the state vocational rehabilitation system. Although this system paid for supports for Kevin's successful college job, it later declared him "unemployable."

Not having a productive job can be as devastating for people with disabilities as it is for their non-disabled peers. Having a disability is expensive, and paying for supports and equipment can eat up a lot of a person's paycheck. But at least if that is earned money coming in, the person has more choices in life than someone who relies on government support. Kevin would like to move out on his own. He has pursued a number of different options, but all have resulted in dead ends from lack of sufficient income.

After fighting with the service systems that support people with physical disabilities for so long, and not finding the support Kevin needed to move out or get another job, Carl, Kevin, and I eventually made the agonizing decision to apply to the Department of Mental Retardation. Our state has a self-determination program which allows people to design their own support system. We hoped that Kevin would be able to find more housing and employment services by going this route. So Kevin was tested and accepted as a client of DMR. As a result, he is on waiting lists for employment and residential services. Both of these waiting lists contain literally thousands of names. And because Kevin is now able to receive services through DMR (at least in theory) he is ineligible for any other services offered to people with physical disabilities. Forget about falling through the cracks. We are living in the hole underneath the cracks!

We have been fighting the system for so long, and we continue to fight the system, but we aren't winning. So we as a family have begun focusing our attention elsewhere.

Kevin's brother Jason works at a nearby Easter Seal camp, and suggested that Kevin volunteer there one or two days a week. Jay made the arrangements through his friends, and Kevin has been there for about two years. It has been great. He is with people who like him, want to be with him, and are not paid to be with him. They choose to be there, and that makes all the difference. Through this job, Kevin met Ed, a retired man who works in the housekeeping area. Ed is a man of many talents, and he enjoys making devices for people with disabilities out of wood and metal. Ed had never known someone with a disability before he met Kevin. But because of Kevin, Ed has become quite a resource for people around here.

We have become involved with a campground where we spend our weekends from April to November. When we first drove in there, we just had a feeling that this would be a good place for us. The whole campground is completely flat, and pretty accessible. When you go up to the office, there are little ramps to get you in. So Kevin can go all around by himself. I am an introvert; I would rather stay at the trailer with a few close friends. Kevin is an extrovert; he goes all over the camp talking with everybody. If he needs me, he calls me on the walkie-talkie. Then at the end of the day, we go for a walk together and all we hear from one end of the campground to the other is "Hey, Kevin!" "What's up, Kev?" "Hey, it's great to see you!" I wonder, how do all these people know Kevin? But that is who he is: a very sociable person.

So we have two or three days on the weekend that are happy; and we have one or two days during the week that are happy. We focus on that. We have to. Someday we hope that the service system will be able to provide Kevin with what he needs to live a full life in the community. In the meantime, it is important that we enjoy the life we have right now.

For many years, Pat Beeman has been an outspoken advocate for people with disabilities and others who are overlooked in our fast-paced society. In the summer of 2000, Pat lost her voice for about six weeks due to a viral infection. She was not sick – she was at The Community Place every day – but she was just unable to speak. Seeing for herself how people with communication issues are treated had a profound effect on Pat. In the midst of her silence, she typed out some thoughts about this experience. As we have mentioned earlier, people's gifts may be obscured by their disabilities; but more often, the failure lies in our ability to perceive those gifts, and to understand that we are more alike than we realize.

LESSONS FROM SILENCE
Pat Beeman

Here are some beginnings of the things I have learned. It is my hope that someday there will be more of an appreciation of how much we need communication in our lives. A small thing like "voice" is something which should not be taken lightly. I also hope that when we see someone in our midst who does not communicate through "voice" -- it could be a person who doesn't know our language, or someone who is deaf, or someone who speaks in a manner other than the usual physical voice – there will be compassion and understanding. There will be thought given about how to make this person feel a part of things instead of feeling left out. There will be new ways to say "you are of value," "I embrace you," and "your opinion matters."

"Not being able to speak does not mean I don't have anything to say." Many of us have seen that statement on T-shirts, posters, and post cards, but it has never rung as true to me as it has during this time. How am I now able to function as a valued human being? How can I perform my job as manager of a post office and card/gift/book store? How do my employees react to this condition? What do the customers do? How do the "regulars" respond when I try to have a surface conversation with them (but really can't without my voice)? And how do I react to being put into this situation, temporarily having a disability?

It is already difficult to live the SPIRIT of who you are when a physical dimension of your being has been taken away. Other people's reactions amplify this effect. THE VOICE creates camaraderie, surface relationship, a way to get to know another person through small talk... It makes it possible for someone else to know whether you are a kind person or a sarcastic person, all in the way that you interact with your voice. But how does one do the same thing without a voice to rely on?

I write on my noteboard: "I am not rude. I have just lost my voice." The reactions vary:

- "Where did it go?"
- "Silence is Golden."
- "I'm sorry to hear that."
- "This is a blessing for you."
- One person begins singing lines from the old Simon and Garfunkel song, *Sounds of Silence*: "Hello darkness my old friend..."
- One person gives me a hug.
- Some try to use humor, such as "Will you speak up?" or "I haven't read this much in a long time."
- Some ask me a question, but instead of waiting for me to write down the answer, say "Forget it" and leave abruptly.
- Some people think it is a joke.
- Some become silent themselves.
- Others forget they have a voice, and start answering my scribbled notes by writing down their responses.
- Three of us are standing together talking (I'm writing). When we part, one person says goodbye to the other, but not to me. She just walks away, forgetting that I even exist because now I don't have a voice.
- Someone cries in front of me. I listen to her issues and try to console her. But she doesn't have time to read my words of encouragement. In this circumstance, people tend to be more

abrupt than appreciative as I try to support them. A hug does help, but it is only part of the answer.

♦ Some grow impatient while I write. One lady needs to put on her glasses before she can read. She resents this so much that I have to go and find an interpreter.

♦ My employee says, "It takes too long working with you. The line at the cash register is getting too long. I need to get someone else in to help us out."

I have a host of emotions in response to these experiences. I feel lonely and frustrated. I am left out of conversations, or feel as if I am in the way. I want to scream because people go away so abruptly. On the other hand, some people talk on and on, and I have so much I want to say to them. My mind is so full of thoughts that I grow too tired to write down every nuance and expression.

Sometimes I need to find an interpreter to explain what I am trying to say, or to make phone calls. What a disaster. That is when I become most frustrated because people do not relay the information in the manner I want the listener to receive it. When those I work with won't explain my situation to customers, people look at me as if I am rude.

I have learned that it takes a bright, intuitive individual to transmit the SPIRIT part of me. We live in such a physical world. People are not in touch with the spiritual; and learning from the body, mind, and spirit as a "whole" does not come easily to us. It helps if someone is willing to learn a little about who I am to break the ice. It also helps if people try to make me a part of things, rather than treating me as if I am a nuisance.

In general, people won't TAKE THE TIME TO LISTEN (in whatever form that is), or when they do my spirit comes out in tomes of pages. One day I was helping a dad who was trying to find something to say to his daughter who had just gotten engaged. It was a stimulating conversation, but hard because I had tons of things to say but not the energy to write it all down. I get tired of doing it this way, and missing the opportunity to make my point because it just takes too much energy.

I find myself alone in this process, trying to feel my way through, trying to figure out how to communicate my emotions, my spirit, and my frustrations. I want someone to cry with me, laugh with me, listen to me, understand me, and not make fun of me. I want help in getting to know who Pat is without a voice.

Naturally, there is a difference between having been born with a disability versus receiving a disability from accident or circumstance. There is also a difference between saying "She can't speak" and "She has lost her voice." These two descriptions bring out distinct reactions from people. I prefer "She has lost her voice" because many people have lost their ability to talk at one time or another. They know what it feels like. But when described as unable to speak, people cannot relate to the experience. They feel sorry for me and step back, increasing my sense of isolation.

I find it hard not to remember myself as I had been. I am forced to live in the present moment because the past is gone. I have to stop thinking "if only" I could say this or that. I want to say so much, but I can't right now. But if I could sit down with people and spend time with them, we might be able to understand one another.

I feel I must spend too much energy explaining myself and defending myself. Couldn't people just take me as I am? When someone puts me at ease and allows me to be myself, that is when I feel the difference. I begin to feel respected. I begin to feel that I still belong.

There are a few individuals who make me feel better. They take time with me, and really want to read my notes. They respond with their voices. They try to understand my pain rather than brushing me off. They have a conversation with me in the normal way, not making me feel like a freak.

Several of these sensitive people have said they felt touched by things I have written to them; but I am unsure whether these things, if said out loud, would have had the same impact. Somehow there have been times when I have affected people more without my voice than with it. Recently, I explained (in writing) my frustration to someone I know is a kind individual. She gave me a hug and went away saying, "I have learned something today."

In the end, so have I.

AND SOMETIMES YOU DO…

After I moved out on my own, Pat Beeman asked me to write several articles about how things were going. The first time, I looked at her in disbelief because she had been walking with me through all of the difficulties and tears. She knew this would not be a happy tale. "I don't think I can write about *that*," I said. "It has been so hard! People want to hear about how well everything has turned out… I don't want to make them sad or frightened." Pat replied, "People want to know the truth. Just write about things the way they are." So I wrote two articles which turned out to be among the most popular we ever ran in our newsletter.

Some of us are able to cope with adversity in a graceful manner, but that does not mean everything is going smoothly. From sharing my struggles, whether privately with a friend or publicly through writing or speaking, I have learned how much strength people draw from one another's experiences. Whenever I have described what I thought was my own weakness in a situation, I have been surprised at the reaction. Every time, people have said, "Thanks so much for telling me about this. I feel so much better knowing that you find it difficult too." If I have been able to help them by talking about my experiences, I am glad. Their words of acceptance and appreciation have been a gift to me as well.

REACHING YOUR DREAM IS ONLY HALF THE BATTLE
Cathy Ludlum

It took five years for me to become a member of a housing cooperative. This journey was shared with a group of friends who became my circle of support. On February 3, after endless delays and disappointments, my dream came true as I moved into the Common Thread Housing Co-op in Manchester, Connecticut.

In this article I want to include the many victories of this year: being elected president of our 16-family complex; learning to juggle cooking, cleaning, and related household tasks; increasing my ability to stay by myself; surviving a cold (not ever a sure thing); and continuing to get the support I need from my circle members, roommates, assistants, neighbors, and friends. I also want to mention what my mother is doing these days, how she bought a little red car and, for the first time in 29 years, truly has a life of her own.

But that is only half the story. To say that everything is wonderful now would be to deny the personal trauma involved in any transition and the inevitable change a dream undergoes as it becomes a reality.

During the first few weeks, people kept saying, "Your dream has come true! You must be so excited." Actually, I alternated between being numb and being terrified. Everything was so different, and I had so many new responsibilities. Most of the things which were familiar to me were still in boxes, and I was constantly in need of things I didn't yet have (a plunger, a sharp knife, scotch tape). I was too overwhelmed to think about buying curtains or hanging pictures, so I left the walls bare and relied on the white shades that came with the windows.

Then there were all the problems inherent in moving into a brand new building; handles came off of doors, hot water was either too hot or non-existent, a pipe in the bathroom leaked under the wall and into my bedroom. Gradually, things were repaired and personal touches started appearing in my new space; but it was many, many weeks before I started to feel comfortable here.

In addition to the natural stress of the situation, there were more practical concerns. The support system my circle and I had designed called for me to share my three-bedroom unit with two live-in assistants. Lisa and I moved in hoping that we would find our third person soon. For three months, we tried and failed to recruit a suitable person. In the meantime, we got up at 5:00 a.m. so Lisa could get me ready and be on the road to her full-time job by 8:00. We survived with the help of friends and part-time people, but everyone involved experienced a certain amount of exhaustion and frustration.

It was much harder for me to manage time effectively with my assistants and to get everything done. I had been hiring assistants for several years while living with my mother, but if I forgot something or ran short of time, she was there to tie up the loose ends. Now, I had so much more to do that I couldn't even think of tasks in three-hour segments. On occasion, I had to decide between eating and going to the bathroom because there was not time to do both, plus buy food, cook it, and still keep up with my job. I hired more people to work more hours, and my savings account shrank alarmingly.

Beyond the personal struggles, our whole co-op was going through its own growing pains. We all moved in during a two-week period, so everyone was in a state of transition at the same time. Tempers were short and often people walked around looking tired and upset.

We hadn't yet finished our house rules (a document developed by each co-op to govern the details of our shared lives), so we didn't have guidelines to deal with some of the situations that came up.

An issue which surfaced early and continues to haunt us is the role people with disabilities should play in maintaining the co-op. As resident/owners, all occupants must participate actively in the management and upkeep of the property. Those of us with disabilities (a lawyer, a tax expert, a writer, and a former salesman) could not really mow grass effectively, but believed we would be able to contribute in other ways that were of equal value.

Through a complicated series of events, however, the co-op decided that administrative work doesn't count toward our 2-hour-a-month maintenance requirement. Instead, the general feeling is that our maintenance responsibilities should be waived or performed by our spouses or roommates. Although we do feel accepted in the co-op, to make physical maintenance a primary requirement of residency is to put those of us who cannot perform it in an uncomfortable position. We are not in danger of punitive action, but neither are we allowed to contribute to the co-op according to our individual talents and have it counted as maintenance. No solution has yet been found, but we keep trying.

One of the hardest things to accept is that "community" has a negative aspect as well as the positive ones we always talk about. It is where ALL people belong, and it is worth fighting to see people included, but that does not mean it is always pleasant.

Along with the spontaneity, the naturalness of relationships, the fun, the strength, and the creativity, there is also the tendency to form cliques, to make judgements, to start rumors, to get in one another's way, to make enemies as well as friends. People have had personal struggles which have affected everyone in the co-op. There are many children living here, and it is sometimes difficult to supervise them adequately. Pets, parking, and use of the community room have also caused contention among us.

This shouldn't surprise those of us who had the vision, but somehow it does. There is a sadness associated with the loss of the perfect little neighborhood which existed only in our minds. That is not to say we could have or would have done anything differently. Instead, it is an acknowledgement of the difference between a dream and a reality.

And I am perhaps overstating the problems. Those of us who live here have reached our dreams in various ways.

Some of us came to the co-op seeking safety. I have called on my neighbors to say that I needed assistance with breathing, and they have rushed right over. Other members wanted a secure environment in which to raise their children; they came here to escape substandard housing, drugs, or crime. They too, have found what they were looking for. We all watch each other's homes, cars, and kids, and anyone who would harm one of us would have to contend with all of us.

Some came in search of a true neighborhood. In spite of the problems, people do hang out together in the courtyard, and eat dinner in one another's homes. We have been able to rely on one another for rides, for car repairs, for help in carrying things, and in countless other situations. There have been joint shopping trips. We held an Easter egg hunt for the children, worked together to plan the dedication of our co-op, and on the Fourth of July most of us went to the same fireworks display.

Things have improved greatly in the last six months, and the more we iron out the bugs, the better it will be.

I am increasingly happy to be living here. As I get settled, I become more able to interact with the members of the co-op and be involved in the town of Manchester. It's getting easier to juggle the responsibilities of my support system, house, and job. My circle is encouraging me to make time for myself (now, there's a thought!). I am beginning to hang pictures on my walls, and to consider painting parts of my unit something other than white.

Best of all, my dread of ending up in a nursing home recedes further and further into the background as that possibility becomes more remote. Life is hard sometimes, but we are coping. My dream was not that my life be made easy or perfect, but that my ability to live the way I want to live remain intact far into the future.

This is what has happened ... and what is *really* worth getting excited about!

This story is adapted from an article in the *Communitas Communicator*, Vol. 3, No. 3, Fall 1992.

SETTLING IN
Cathy Ludlum

It has been almost two years since I moved from my mother's home into a housing cooperative. While this represents a great victory, there is another side to the story which I neither anticipated nor recognized until recently. At this point, I would like to share some of the patterns I've been noticing in the hope that they will be helpful to others undergoing (or enduring?) similar transitions.

Transition Sickness

Watching and participating in the birth of the Common Thread Co-op was great fun in some ways. It was breathtaking to see the progress from March to January, as torn brown earth sprouted foundations, foundations grew up into framed walls, and walls became sealed with brick and with glass. Finally, the addition of cabinets and appliances signaled the approach of moving day.

Unfortunately, my enjoyment of the process was interrupted by a series of colds, upset stomachs, and bad asthma attacks, which started in early October. For nearly four months, I was sick more often than I was well, and I even spent two weeks in the hospital with pneumonia. I was sick on Election Day, I was sick on Christmas, and I was so sick on New Year's Eve that I nearly returned to the hospital. But with the help of many friends, I remained at home until that episode passed ten days later.

Now, you need to understand that I never get sick. I get one cold every year, and that's it. To my mother and all my friends, it was obvious that I was reacting to my upcoming move, but it wasn't at all obvious to me. The only thing I knew was that I had felt lousy for months. Then, just when it seemed like my body would never be the same again, I became able (finally) to breathe and to eat.

And just in time! Three weeks later I moved.

Frantic, Numb, and Exhausted

So here I was, in my own home that I'd dreamed of and fought for such a long time. Was I excited? Actually, *frantic, numb, and exhausted* described it better. I had expected the move to be stressful, but the mental and physical strain was more significant and lasted far longer than I could have guessed. I moved in on February 3, and didn't truly start to relax until Thanksgiving.

During this time, I tried to function as normally as possible, going to work, coordinating my personal assistants, and trying to keep up with housework, bills, food shopping, cooking, and so on. But I felt completely overwhelmed most of the time. It was difficult to concentrate; I was plagued by unexpected and unexplained tears; I tended to snap at people who called because I didn't think I could handle one more thing. Although these problems decreased over time, they persisted for almost a year. Thankfully, my first housemate, Lisa, and my other friends and circle members were understanding and supportive at all times.

The circle was always there with offers of help – to run errands, make phone calls, make schedules – but to some extent, the feelings were separate from the circumstances. I was never really caught up, but catching up was not the issue. I was in a strange place, trying to carry on as if nothing had changed. While help was needed and appreciated, I just had to live through this period, and there was no way to live through it any faster.

Making Mistakes

How would I find my live-in assistants? How much would their services cost? Would I be able to juggle everything that needed juggling? Could I really afford to live on my own? The jury's still out on some of these, but my circle and I have always known how much we didn't know about my new life, and decided that the first few years would be spent making mistakes and learning from them.

By now, I've made lots of mistakes and done some learning. I've learned why you don't put regular dish detergent in the dishwasher, and what catfish tastes like when you haven't cooked it long enough. I've learned to expect surprises, and to allow people to help me cope with them. I've learned the importance of sharing my dreams with potential housemates upfront, so our dreams don't come into conflict later on. I've learned about compromise, but I've also learned that I don't always have to be the one to give in.

On the other hand, my books don't balance yet; I haven't found a reliable way of recruiting new live-in assistants; and I continue to have difficulty coordinating my time commitments so that I can eat and sleep sufficiently. I still don't look in my mailbox every day, and have occasionally paid late fees on bills or had to write letters of apology to the IRS (guess I wrote a good letter though, because the IRS refunded my penalty!).

Getting Settled

By the one-year mark, I actually began to feel like I knew what I was doing. I paid bills when they arrived; planned two "cooking days" a week, rather than trying to cook something every day; and made it a priority to attend a singles fellowship once a week no matter how busy I was. I started trying not to work on weekends. I was more comfortable being alone, and changed my support system from two live-in assistants to one.

As more months passed, I became able to look beyond the daily details, to think about making my unit more cozy and my life more fun. Friends made curtains for my living-room, dining room, and kitchen, and painted my walls. This summer I unpacked all those books that had been sitting in boxes for 18 months, and spent a week at a retreat center in New Hampshire. I even acquired a pet, a little green and orange ("sherbet colored") lovebird named Sherbie. I don't have lots of time to spare, but am trying to make it a priority to sit quietly, and to read books that are not about disability issues. This semester I will be taking a language class on Monday nights, and am setting aside some time for homework.

There is an increasing sense of well-being in my life. Although it is punctuated by minor crises, my circle and I have developed many strategies to return me to a state of normalcy. My optimism about the future increases almost daily.

As I have gone through all these stages, I have discovered that there is no such thing as "moving day." Moving (or any major transition) takes place, not in days or weeks, but in years. My two-year anniversary in the co-op will be February 3, and I think I am now, finally, all moved in!

This story was adapted from a two-part series in the *Communitas Communicator*, Vol. 4, No.3, Fall 1993; and Vol. 4, No. 4, Winter 1993.

For years, Pat and George had talked about starting a diner. They envisioned a place where the things we were learning about community (the importance of shared meals, conversation, time together) could be put into practice. Eventually, they did start a business in downtown Manchester, but it was not a restaurant. It was – and is – a unique combination of merchandise and philosophy. And they discovered that community has its problems as well as its advantages.

THE COMMUNITY PLACE:
MORE THAN A PLACE, A WAY OF WELCOMING
George Ducharme and Pat Beeman

"Building Positive and Inclusive Communities" is the mission statement of Communitas, and The Community Place is the visible expression of this concept.

Communitas opened The Community Place to demonstrate one path to a positive and inclusive community. Located on Main Street in Manchester, Connecticut, it is so much more than a gift shop. Everything from the automatic door; the wider-than-usual aisles; the placement of cards, gifts, and books; to the deliberate selection of diverse ethnic and cultural images shows that this is a place where *all* are truly welcome. At The Community Place, the gifts of each person are respected, appreciated, and supported.

In a corner of the store is the Gathering Space, a cherished dining room table where people come together for tea, classes, conversation, and meetings. Surrounded by colorful posters and interesting books, the space gives community a place to happen. People with disabilities and all excluded people know the results of negative communities. But the circle of friends who come to the Gathering Space are working slowly and persistently to transform negative attitudes into something more welcoming. The mission of Communitas, particularly for Pat, Bev, and George, is to help the people in our part of the community to be more open toward all people who are different. The cards and gifts, along with the events at the Gathering Space bring people together in a circle of support. This circle is not a formal entity, but a connection which occurs naturally every day and every place.

This circle widens to include the people who provide the labor and the environment which provides the raw materials of the products we sell. For we cannot push to include our friends with disabilities into community life if we do not also respect and appreciate all people and our planet itself. This adds yet another dimension to our work, but we feel it is essential. All people are "gifted," and we need to support one another in creating a world where justice and peace prevail.

It seems like an impossible task for a small struggling store in the downtown district of a medium-sized New England town. Still, we work toward building a positive and inclusive *community* because we think this is the next step toward making a world which accepts the gifts of all people.

Pat and George are writing a book about their experiences at The Community Place. For more information, contact them at Communitas, P. O. Box 358, Manchester, CT 06045-0358 USA or call 860-645-6976.

WHAT HAPPENS WHEN YOU GET THERE...

CIRCLE MAINTENANCE

Circles of support are a great tool, but like other tools, they present both opportunities and limitations. The opportunities have been well-publicized, and those of us who believe in the circle concept are always eager to share success stories. In this section, however, we would like to outline some of the realities involved with doing a circle.

Circles are a lot of work – A circle can be of great benefit to people, but it does not start by itself, and it will die out if it is not maintained. To keep a circle going, someone needs to set meeting dates, notify circle members, arrange a location, and arrange for followup activities. Taking notes is helpful, and having snacks at the meeting is traditional, though not absolutely necessary. The irony is that the higher the level of stress in a person's life, the less likely he or she will be to pull all this together. If a member of the circle is willing to invite the other members, this is often enormously helpful.

Circles work best when there is a clear vision – When a person has a clear vision of the future, the circle has concrete activities to perform and people tend to be motivated to join in. Once the goal has been accomplished (for example, the person has moved into the new home), there is no longer a specific goal to rally around. The circle may go through a crisis of inertia. If the circle is to continue, additional goals should be identified. They may be targeted toward addressing new crises (the person is living on his or her own, but needs additional support). Or, if things are going well, new activities might focus on getting more connected in the community or having recreational opportunities.

Circles are sometimes time-limited, and this is okay – Keeping a circle going forever may be useful, or it may be a source of additional stress. Each person or family will decide whether the benefits outweigh the work involved. A circle can be disbanded and reconvened at a later time. It is critical, however, that maintaining relationships be an ongoing priority. Friends and neighbors make life more fun, they may be needed for support in the future, and it is important to be of support to them so relationships do not become one-way.

INCLUSION AND RELIGION

In the late 1980s, when we began using the One Candle Power methods in Connecticut, we believed that religious people and organizations would be natural allies in welcoming people with disabilities. In some circumstances, this has certainly been the case. People from the congregation have volunteered to drive a member with a disability to church on Sundays, or invited a participant for Sabbath lunch after synagogue services. There are many stories of people being fully included in their religious communities.

Unfortunately, this level of acceptance has not been universal. People – even religious people – often carry the same stereotypes as the rest of the general population. Some misconceptions may have a distinctly spiritual theme; for example, when my friend asked her new priest about making the building wheelchair accessible, he responded that she did not need to be in church anyway because she could not sin. Though unintentional, a coldness toward people who are perceived as different has made full participation in religious life seem like a distant dream.

For some people with disabilities and their families, this is fine. They may not choose a spiritual path for themselves; or if they do, they prefer to follow it alone.

If you desire a religious connection, there are a number of ways to pursue that goal.

> I want to be thoroughly used up when I die, for the harder I work, the more I live. I rejoice in life for its own sake. Life is no "brief candle" to me. It is a sort of splendid torch which I have got hold of for a moment, and I want to make it burn as brightly as possible before handing it on to future generations.
>
> George Bernard Shaw

Try different congregations – Congregations are like people: each one has its own strengths, weaknesses, personality, and quirks. It may take some time to find a good match.

Look for good listeners – People who want to fix everything are often uncomfortable with people with disabilities. Try to find people who see this situation as an opportunity for them to learn something, and not just as a way to help someone they think of as "less fortunate."

Make one connection, and watch it grow – If you can connect with one person in a congregation, and have that person see you for who you really are, you have found something priceless. Enjoy the friendship as it develops. At the right time, this person will introduce you to others in that faith community.

Remember that not all spiritual people do "organized religion" – While churches, synagogues, and other religious institutions offer an opportunity for people to meet and socialize, there are many people who prefer alternate paths. Meditation classes, social action groups, and other activities also draw people who are interested in making the world a better place. If something appeals to you, go and try it. You never know who might be waiting to meet you!

A few years ago, I became dissatisfied with my spiritual identity. My decision to convert to Judaism took many people by surprise, including the members of my circle, but it is a journey which started 25 years ago. In the story that follows, I describe this journey.

MATTERS OF FAITH
Cathy Ludlum

I have always been a spiritual person. I remember being five years old and thinking about God, but having no real focus for my thoughts. At the age of 14 I became a born-again Christian, and was excited to have a framework I could use to think about spiritual things. I began to read the Bible for myself, and for the first time fully realized that Jesus was Jewish. So, while still in high school, I began to study Hebrew. I hoped someday to be able to read the Scriptures in their original language.

For almost 20 years, Christianity was a strong part of my identity. In college, I participated in Campus Crusade for Christ, where I made many friends. Through this group, I had my first opportunity to go on weekend retreats. These were wonderful times. Later, I was involved with several small evangelical churches. The best years were in a church in Manchester, where I was completely accepted and my gifts were sought out by many of the members. I became immersed in a singles group, and am still in touch with several people I met there.

But there was always something missing… Although I loved both of the churches I attended over the years, I never felt compelled to take the next step toward membership, which involved taking classes and making a formal commitment to the church. Somehow I had not yet found the right fit. I had a vague awareness that much of the Jewish heritage had been washed out of Christianity, and somehow this bothered me. What had happened to Passover? What had happened to the Sabbath? There were so many holy days mentioned in the Bible. Weren't they important anymore? Why were Jewish prophets given so little attention compared to New Testament teachers? And, being a Christian, why did it matter to me? I felt this way even before Stephen came into my life, but our friendship caused me to examine these issues more closely.

Stephen and I first met at my job. For a while, I dreaded seeing him; our perspectives were so different that it was hard for us to hold a conversation. Eventually, a friendship did develop, but still we didn't seem to connect very well. Then, one Christmas, I sent Stephen a holiday letter with a strong Christian slant. I sent a similar letter every year to about 80 of my closest friends, including Jews, and as far as I knew no one had ever been offended by it. So I was surprised when Stephen called to complain. I explained that the letter was meant to share who I was and what I'd been doing during the year, and was not intended as criticism of anyone else. Once Stephen calmed down and we really began to talk, we realized we had an extraordinary amount in common.

Stephen, too, was very spiritual, and because of his Judaism we shared many of the same values. He was amazed by how much I knew about the Hebrew Scriptures, and I was interested in how he interpreted them, even though his interpretations seemed odd to me. We talked about growing up in Sunday school and Hebrew School; about the cultural bias against things spiritual; and about discrimination, history, and prophecy. It was a stimulating series of conversations, and I wanted to continue them. From knowing Stephen, I was finally getting to see Judaism first-hand.

I learned the basics of keeping kosher, at first in an effort to feed Stephen when he came to visit. But I was always conscious that Jesus observed the Jewish dietary laws, and wondered whether I shouldn't try also. Gradually, I gave up bacon and shellfish, and finally meat altogether. It isn't necessary to become vegetarian in order to keep kosher, but it makes things easier.

Later, as Stephen began observing Shabbat (the Jewish Sabbath), I started trying to incorporate a rest day into my schedule. It wasn't easy; there was always so much that had to get done. But I started small. I chose one Saturday, and spent the whole day listening to sermons and music on tape. I felt so much better afterward that I decided to try to reserve Saturday as a spiritual day, to study, write, and pray. Later, I began taking Friday night as well, and lighting a candle to focus my attention. When Stephen put a message on his answering machine asking not to be disturbed from Friday evening at sundown until Saturday evening at sundown, I thought this was a spectacular idea and put a similar message on my machine. This was probably the best move of all. So much of my stress is associated with the phone (personal assistants calling in sick, my endless work calls, etc.), and I have developed a dislike of hearing it ring.

Everything came to a screeching halt when I began to formally join a "Jews for Jesus" style congregation. While for me this represented a perfect blend of everything I thought I wanted – Christianity and Judaism together – most Jews considered it a hideous concept. Stephen and I had had numerous debates about who Jesus was, as well as about

Biblical prophecy, Christian antisemitism, and the role of faith vs. deeds. But we always managed to remain friends in spite of our differences. Now that I was officially becoming associated with this group, the rhetoric on both sides heated up considerably. Then Stephen attended a talk by a representative from a counter-missionary organization, and brought over a handful of booklets which he dared me to read. I have never subscribed to the view that you shouldn't read certain things. I believed then, and still believe now, that it's what you don't know that can hurt you.

I found the materials surprisingly convincing. I struggled to defend what i thought was the truth, but the arguments I used seemed less compelling than what I was reading. Although this process took only three days, it was many months before I could say out loud that I wasn't a Christian anymore. In the meantime, I moaned to Stephen that I was no longer the same person. He asked some questions intended to show me that although my frame of reference had shifted, the real "me" (whatever that means) had not changed. For the next five months, I tried to salvage any parts of Christianity that I could still use, but the spell was broken. I didn't believe it anymore.

Then came the process of figuring out where I belonged spiritually. It took a long time, but when I looked back at my religious history and interests, the direction my life had been going was already pretty clear. There were many similarities between my old spiritual style and my new one in terms of values, commitment to family, emphasis on prayer and study of the Scriptures, and connecting with God in every moment of life. Still uncertain, however, I spent eight weeks visiting synagogues in what I called "the synagogue experiment." Everywhere I went I was warmly welcomed, and by then I knew enough about the service to feel somewhat comfortable. So I began the process of conversion.

Every major decision we make in life affects not only us, but also the people closest to us. As I changed from a Christian perspective to a Jewish one, the members of my circle shared my initial loss, my exploration of options, and my emergence into a new stage of my life. In the beginning, some were concerned that Stephen was having too much of an influence over me. Most realized that my interest in Judaism went way back, and came to share my excitement as I began to embrace the tradition more fully.

My new path has not been particularly smooth. As I have tried to incorporate Jewish practices into my life, my disability has presented a number of challenges. My circle meetings have included many discussions about how I can fit into the Jewish community, both physically and socially. Simply turning pages in a Jewish prayer book has been an obstacle, as I can no longer turn pages for myself. When I have brought a friend or assistant to support me (which I rarely did in the church days because I was stronger then), congregation members have tended to hang back. Perhaps they have not known how to relate to me, or maybe they have seen me as self-sufficient because I had a helper. I have felt drawn to a synagogue where the people are friendly, but the building has major accessibility problems, and my circle and I have held brainstorming sessions about how to reduce the barriers. I am getting there, but it is taking time, as everything does.

My circle has existed for over fifteen years now. People have married and divorced, had babies, struggled with teenagers, changed careers, bought and sold homes, and lost loved ones. Life, with its rhythm of joy and sorrow and change, continues for each member of the circle, and for all of us together as a kind of extended family. My decision to change from Christian to Jew may have been unique; but my circle continues to be the accepting, nurturing base from which I can dare to dream.

MIXED BLESSINGS AND MIXED SIGNALS

We all work hard to establish relationships, and hope that people will truly become a part of our lives. We look forward to the day when our new friends will call us up and ask us to the movies, or out to eat, or to their home to play with their cat.

Time goes by, and suddenly we are bombarded by phone calls and invitations. We are frightened. We are upset. We say no. Or we say yes, but we worry the whole time we are out.

What happened?

It could be any number of things: fear of the unknown, shyness, uncertainty about how to behave.

For people with severe physical disabilities, spontaneity is a problem. This is difficult to explain to well-intentioned community folks. If people are scheduled to come in at a specific time to act as formal (paid) supports, it is not a good idea to cancel or dramatically change their schedule at the last minute. Like any other job, people expect to start at a specific time. People with physical disabilities may also have to do certain things at certain times (like eating or using the bathroom), and often these activities take longer than they would for someone without physical limitations.

One parent described it this way: "She called up after 3:00 and offered to meet my son at the game if I could drop him off at 5:00. It sounded like such a wonderful opportunity. I didn't want to say no, but I was panicked because now I didn't know what to do about dinner. I was planning to prepare a meatloaf for all of us, but now my son needed to eat earlier. I am diabetic, so I need to eat right at 5:00, which is when I would be dropping him at the game. And then my husband would be coming in from work, and I was just going to heat up the meatloaf for him. Now I would have to make three separate meals, and it was such a lot of extra work and hassle. But people don't understand, and think I want to keep my son from going out and having fun."

People do not mean to be insensitive to our needs. They just don't understand what our lives are like. We need to find ways of showing our new friends how regimented we must be without making them focus on our differences all over again. We need to educate community people that it is better to call us ahead of time instead of suddenly appearing at the door with concert tickets.

Then, as they are welcoming us, we will be able to welcome them also!

This is a story I wrote about my own struggles to manage my everyday existence.

There are many who are living far below their possibilities because they are continually handing over their individualities to others.

Do you want to be a power in the world?
Then be yourself.
Be true to the highest within your soul
and then allow yourself to be governed by no
customs or conventionalities or arbitrary
man-made rules
that are not founded on principle.

Ralph Waldo Trine

STAYING AFLOAT

Cathy Ludlum

For many years, my dream was to move away from home and live on my own. With the help of many people this was accomplished, and I have been living in a housing cooperative for over ten years now.

On one hand, it has been great to demonstrate that someone with disabilities as significant as mine can live in the community with appropriate support. I actually do have a life: I work for a company I helped start; and I enjoy music, reading, writing, being with people, and doing things outdoors. I also have many dreams for the future. I want to complete my conversion to Judaism, write several more books, visit members of my family who live far away, and see places that are part of my family history. The world which seemed to constrain me when I was in my 20s now seems open to my exploration.

On the other hand, so much freedom does not come without a cost. People tend to think of me as pretty successful and independent. This is true to a point, but the image is misleading unless you can see the rest of the picture. You could say that I live in a boat... and with the support of friends I have navigated this boat down rivers, across lakes, and even along the edge of the ocean. This has given me the opportunity to see many different landscapes and to experience many things. But the distance between me and disaster is only as thick as the bottom of my boat.

For example, I must rely on people to come early in the morning to get me up and dressed, put me into my wheelchair, help me with breakfast, and get me off to work. If the phone rings at 5:00 a.m. and the person says, "Sorry, but my car won't start and the other car isn't available either. I won't be in this morning," my whole day is messed up. At best, it is a frantic chase to find someone who can come quickly to get me up. Then, I must trim my morning routine so I can get finished in time. If things are really bad, I may miss a morning meeting or appointment. Although I have been fortunate with the timing of these problems, my luck cannot hold out forever.

These situations are frustrating, but not life-threatening because I tend to develop many layers of contingency plans. When I am home, I have access to an emergency response system so I can call for help in a crisis. I hire more support people than I need so I will always have people who can fill in for one another. A big part of my backup system involves having a roommate who shares my home, and can be available to help me out in an emergency. While I try not to over-rely on her, it is comforting to know she would be there if other options fail. Even so, people not coming in to work creates an atmosphere of chaos.

In between these disruptions, I am able to enjoy my life. I am involved with many wonderful people, and I am busy trying to make a difference in the world. Most of the time, I feel privileged to be on the cutting edge of changes in the human service system and in our communities. Better times are coming; I can almost taste it.

But there is never one moment of certainty... NOT EVER!

I can be just cruising through my day, and suddenly there is another leak in my boat. The phone rings. My next assistant has come down with strep throat and won't be in tonight. So I drop everything and start calling people to see who can come in. One is on vacation; another has school all evening; another cannot find child care with one hour's notice. Eventually, between paid support people and friends, I am able to patch something together that will at least meet my most basic needs. Out goes the list of things I was planning to do that night with my other assistant. Now that things are resolved, I return to my computer and try to pick up where I left off.

But something is still wrong. My head hurts. My adrenaline is flowing. I feel as if I have brought my boat through strong wind and fierce waves. Although the sky has cleared and the sun is beginning to shine again, my life feels in disarray. Some things on the deck have been washed overboard. Downstairs in the cabin, books and dishes lie scattered on the floor, victims of the rough seas. It is difficult to concentrate in such surroundings, especially knowing that other storms lay ahead, undetected.

What makes it bearable is my circle of support, both my formal circle and my less formal network of friends and fellow travelers. Sometimes I need to call one of my women friends and ask for help with something basic like going to the bathroom. If it is at all feasible for her to come, I know she will; and whether she can come or not she will always say, "Thanks for thinking of me. Call again if I can do anything!" I may have to call six… ten… fourteen people, but so far someone has always come through.

Sometimes in a circle meeting we will brainstorm ways of restructuring staffing patterns to make it easier to find and keep good personal assistants. I am so used to reorganizing my needs to accommodate the preferences of others that I don't even realize what I am doing. It is important to have circle members ask, "So what do YOU want? Don't forget about yourself."

I am about the most optimistic person you will ever meet, but now and then I just need to talk to someone about how hard all this is. One or another of my friends has always been there. She cannot fix everything, but she can listen and understand, and usually that is what I need most.

Every day I feel that I am working hard to stay afloat, yet I intend to keep moving in my little boat. I may be frightened, but as long as I have people who are willing to support my dreams, I can never be content to hide in the shallow water.

Creating the housing cooperative was a very important step in my transition from my mother's home. Moving here and learning to sail and to swim has taught me so much. I have a better sense of my personal capabilities and my capabilities when supported by others. But I did not find the community spirit here that I had hoped for. Although I know my neighbors, making decisions together with them has made it difficult to form true friendships.

So now, after ten years of successful (though bumpy) sailing, I am again rocking the boat. I have decided to buy a house… my own house where I can decide what the yard looks like and where people can park. This is an ambitious undertaking, I realize. It will cost me money, put an additional strain on my support system, and increase the burden of responsibility upon me. This is true of anyone who purchases a home, though, and I feel ready to make the change.

Maybe I am doing the right thing, and maybe I am making a mistake. Either way, it is the beginning of another voyage…

SUPPORT VS. STRANGULATION

One of the balancing acts of One Candle Power is discovering how much support is needed without strangling the person.

I tend to think of this as similar to having a good head-rest. Ever since I was fourteen years old, I have not been able to hold my head up without support. While I have been offered many head-rests which would hold the head in a vice-like grip, I would never allow such a thing to be mounted on my wheelchair. I cannot move much, but I want the option of using what movement I still have! Recently, I found something which gives just a little support at the back of my head, with two small wings that jut forward on either side. I am free to move my head as much as I am able; but if I go too far and lose my balance, the side wings keep my head from falling into an uncomfortable position.

In the same way, my friends may offer help or advice; but they are willing to support me in whatever path I may choose for myself. We respect one another's right to autonomy, even when we do not agree. If I fall into a hole, my friends are there to pull me out. And if they fall into a hole, I am there for them as well.

And as we support one another, we continue to grow in our friendships.

I felt incredibly guilty about having another ambitious dream after living in the co-op for just five years. Nevertheless, the pull toward a new stage of my life was irresistible.

THE NEXT DREAM... AND THE NEXT!

Cathy Ludlum

Do people with disabilities have the right to dream? My whole life resonates with the answer: YES!

On a March evening in 1987, my friends committed themselves to making my dream of living on my own come true. The housing cooperative I live in, as well as the organization that developed it, grew out of my vision and the commitment of these people. To say that the work of creating Common Thread Co-op was monumental would be an understatement. It took five years of meetings – breakfast meetings with powerful people, town meetings that went until midnight, Board meetings, finance meetings, architectural meetings, planning meetings – and visits to potential sites to make the co-op a reality. If you have ever built a house; and know of all the delays, pitfalls, and headaches that involves; multiply it by the 16 units in our complex, and you will have a sense of what we went through. At the same time, it took a huge amount of work, on my part and on the part of my friends and family, to prepare me for my new life.

Since 1992, I have lived out my dream of living on my own. I have done this with the support of roommates, personal assistants, and a large network of friends, neighbors, co-workers, and fellow travelers. My co-op unit is beautiful, accessible, and close to shopping and the highway. My friends have helped me paint the rooms – gray-blue in the office, melon-orange in the hall, and robin's egg blue in the bathroom! – even when they thought my color choices were a little strange. Between my ever changing support system and the dynamics of the co-op, things rarely run smoothly. But for the most part I am safe and happy with my life.

I have dreamed the impossible dream and seen it come true. So it seems almost disloyal to say I now want to live somewhere else. Why do I feel that way?

People without disabilities take for granted that they will work in various jobs during their lives, that they will live in different places, pursue dreams, accomplish them, and then move on to new heights. Should not the same standard apply to those of us with disabilities? My head says, of course it should. But my gut, which is very much into not inconveniencing others, and being grateful for everything I get, is having a hard time with the next step.

When I first realized that the center of my life had shifted away from Manchester, and was waiting for me in West Hartford, I was horrified. For ten years, during the five years it took to develop the co-op and for five years after I moved in, I believed that I would live here for the rest of my life. The shift did not happen all at once, but resulted from many other changes. It started with my decision to convert to Judaism. I began attending services in West Hartford, and became intrigued by the rule that worshipers live within walking distance of their synagogue. What at first seemed like an unreasonable demand, eventually began to look like a beautiful way to encourage community.

Once I actually considered the possibility of moving, other advantages came to mind. Some were as mundane as having a shorter commute to work and to concerts I attend in the summer, or living in the same phone district as several people I talk with constantly. Other reasons for moving were more momentous. I had learned how much work it takes to keep a co-op operating, and after five years I wanted to focus my energy differently. I had learned that a sense of community does not automatically flow from having neighbors close by. This was disappointing, but it gave me the urge to keep looking. At the same time, I felt very fortunate to have lived in such a good situation. I had met people whose circumstances were similar to what mine were ten years ago, and who would give anything to live here. Perhaps it was just time for me to move on.

When I timidly mentioned to a few people that I was thinking about buying a house, I was afraid they would feel that their self-sacrifice for the co-op was in vain. Instead they said, in different ways, that we all grow out of things and dream new dreams. They are excited, and eager to walk with me as I reach for the stars yet again.

Even so, it is with a great deal of self-consciousness that I pursue the next stage of my life. Perhaps I feel differently because the urgency of this journey is less intense. It was easy to speak out the last time, to cry out that my mother was getting older and I didn't want to spend my life in a nursing home. But now the issue is not one of physical survival. Can I really move just because I want to, or is this too much of a luxury?

The answer may lie in distancing myself from my own insecurities. If my friend with a disability came to me and said, "My friends and I worked very hard to make my dream happen. Now I want something else. Do I have the right to dream another dream?" I know what I would say to her: "You absolutely do! And anyone who cares about you will be happy to see you grow to this new stage in your life."

Adapted from the Fall, 1999 issue of the *Communitas Communicator.*

Hope is not a guarantee of complete satisfaction. It is a kind of inner power to believe that life can get better, not perfect, just better than it is.

Lewis B. Smedes
Caring and Commitment

MATTERS OF LIFE AND DEATH

Over the course of our lives, we all come into contact with the medical system. Sometimes these exchanges are happy ones, resulting in the birth of a baby or in healing from a serious illness. Unfortunately, for people with disabilities, admission to a hospital often carries its own risks because of stereotypes held by hospital staff.

This section includes the hospital experiences of several people with disabilities. Raymond "Todd" Kilroy was one of the first people in Connecticut to have a circle of support, and his circle stood by him during his struggle with cancer. Circle member Pat Beeman wrote about the time she spent with Todd during his final days.

Next, you will read my own story about a hospital visit which nearly resulted in my death. This was one situation where a circle of support was literally a life-saver!

LESSONS FROM TODD
Pat Beeman

During his lifetime, Raymond "Todd" Kilroy made a difference through his leadership and advocacy on behalf of people with disabilities. In March of 1992, at the age of 55, Todd developed many physical problems which resulted in his death on July 1. His circle walked with him to his death. We helped him to know he was not facing it alone, and he helped us as a circle to face it together. Our lives have been changed, and we have all grown in so many ways. I would like to share these thoughts about some things which made our journey a little easier.

Thanks for Being Here

A number of us in Todd's circle "vigiled" with him through his pain. During one of those times, while he was asleep, I remember thinking to myself, "What am I doing here? I don't seem to be doing anything for him except sitting beside his bed waiting for him to wake up, waiting for him to need me." Todd must have read my mind because just then he woke up out of a deep sleep and asked for his board. He proceeded to spell, "THANKS FOR BEING HERE. IT MEANS A LOT. DON'T WALK AWAY."

Todd taught me more about the importance of "being with" and not always having to be "doing something for" someone. Sometimes that "doing" is just in "being." He taught me that our PRESENCE IN PEOPLE'S LIVES is often the most important gift we can offer.

From Todd I learned that we need to live our lives ONE DAY AT A TIME. We talked a lot about not looking at the past ("What could I have done differently so I didn't get in this situation?"), and not looking to the future ("I won't be able to accomplish what I had planned given my short time to live"). Instead, we must look only at this precious moment, to live fully until we die. What a profound lesson that was for both of us.

Todd and I talked for hours about death, about what it means, what happens, and what to expect. He then fully realized and spelled, "You have no idea how much this talk has meant to me. Thanks for being here. Now, do you know how to play backgammon?" The lesson: okay, we have talked about the reality of what is going to happen, and we have each come to a better understanding of our own mortality. So in the meantime can we have some fun? So the next day I brought in chess games, cards, backgammon, and humor tapes, and we began to live…

Todd taught me the meaning of COMPASSION: "to suffer with." Yes, it is painful, but the joy and healing one can get from facing that pain together is phenomenal. I told Todd, "Life is difficult sometimes, but we want you to know that whatever you have to meet in the months ahead, you will not be facing it alone. We will all meet it with you, no matter what it is." He proceeded to spell, "That means a lot. Thank you for not walking away." And his whole circle got through this with spirit, strength, humor, tears, and pain. But love sustained us through it all.

Compassion is about not walking away, being there for people, suffering in their pain, crying with them, laughing with them, and staying present to them, whatever the cost. There is an incredible enriching of your soul and being that makes you healthier in mind, body, and spirit. It brings forth a resilient and enduring spirit that can help you get through anything. A certain kind of hope remains, even after the person has gone.

I was able to go through the grieving process with Todd. I made my peace with him over the months. We talked about so many different things – things you never get a chance to talk about because there is no time – but I made the time. I was present. I didn't walk away despite the incredible pain I felt at times seeing him suffer. As a circle, we helped Todd face his death together. We all grew; we all celebrated in the presence of each other; we all gave thanks for each new day of breath; and we all sang the symphonies that Todd loved so well.

I learned from Todd's love of Beethoven, that he was much like him. His symphonies go on for hours and they are never finished. So Todd's spirit and vision are with us forever, though his physical presence has died.

May each of us nurture the compassionate presence for others in our lives. Let's continue our walks toward what may lie over the horizon for each of us. Let's grow together through the pain and joy.

Will You See Me for Who I Really Am?

When Raymond "Todd" Kilroy was first admitted to the hospital, we awaited word from doctors as to what might be the problem. A nurse entered the room and asked us very sympathetically, "Has he always suffered like this?" This was a very disturbing question to me. I had never viewed Todd as suffering; on the contrary, he was very active at work, in the community, in advocacy and leadership capacities, and in his church. So I immediately replied to her, "No, he lives a full life in his community in Farmington. He has been sick for some time. Therefore, like anyone else who hasn't been feeling well, he was admitted to do some testing and learn what the problem may be."

This exchange was followed by so many other misconceptions about Todd that I felt the urge to do something. I wanted to find a way for people in the hospital to treat Todd with dignity and respect, to value him as a person and get to know him as we did. But how could people see him for who he was at a time when he was not up to par and could not communicate as he would like?

One Sunday, Beth Mount and I sat with Todd and some large sheets of blank paper. We asked Todd to help us reflect on his life – his interests and hobbies, and the things of which he was most proud – and we added a section for friends to fill in explaining who Todd was to them. As people visited him over many months in various hospitals, the graphic representation of Todd's life sprouted cards and notes describing different memories they had of him. It became a living document of Todd's contributions to the world, and of his personal qualities of sensitivity and graciousness. The charts showed his love of classical music, women, and swimming. As Todd progressively got worse, the document served as a constant reminder to him of his value and dignity as a human being.

The wall charts also became a "bridge" to the doctors, nurses, technicians, and even acquaintances who didn't know Todd well. They began to see him in ways they would never have found if had we not taken the time to write it all down. People in the medical profession began to treat Todd differently. They began to share humor with him, since they now knew that was what he liked; they began to talk about similar interests in classical music, or about places he had been. And as hospital staff, friends, and visitors were "waiting" for procedures to be completed, the chart itself became a topic of conversation.

Later, the nursing staff in the hospice program welcomed the wall charts as a way to see Todd the person instead of Todd the patient. They said that it is very rare for them to see this side of a person when he or she enters hospice.

Todd was truly a man full of talent, humor, love, and ability. I hope this description of these well-used papers bring Todd to life for you as they did for so many during his final days.

Adapted from an article in the *Communitas Communicator*, Vol. 3, No. 3, Fall 1992; and from remarks delivered at his memorial service.

ESCAPE FROM 9 SOUTH *
Cathy Ludlum

[* This is a fictitious hospital unit. What happened to me could have happened anywhere]

Whenever I have gone into the hospital, I have been filled with anxiety. Although most of my hospital experiences have not been too bad, and some have even been positive, I have always been very aware of the risk involved. Let's face it… if you take away my wheelchair and my clothes, I don't look like much. Take away my ability to speak for myself on top of everything else, and I am in actual danger. My body does not react in typical ways. Treatments that might be helpful to a person without a disability may prove deadly for me. Conversely, practices which are not widely accepted are essential to keep me alive.

In 1977, at the age of fourteen, I had pneumonia and landed in the hospital. The medical staff did what they could, but I continued to get worse. I spent three weeks in intensive care, on a ventilator and able to communicate only by writing. I was there so so long that the doctors told my mother the ventilator tube had to be removed from my throat and I would need to have a tracheostomy. Fortunately, she put them off. Meanwhile, I was being given breathing treatments every two hours which included deep suctioning. This involves putting a thin tube through the nose or mouth and all the way down into the large airways in the lungs to literally suck out the mucus. Not only is it uncomfortable… for me, it actually turned out to be harmful.

After a while Dr. Hersh, the resident assigned to my case, suggested that deep suctioning might be irritating my lungs and causing more mucus to form. He gave an order that I not be suctioned anymore. He also taught me, my mother, and all the staff on that floor a technique later called an assisted cough. Pressing down forcefully on my abdomen, he pushed out 21 nasty mucus plugs in our first session. From that day I started to get better.

Dr. Hersh saved my life. And he taught me a mantra which I have used constantly whenever I have been hospitalized: I CANNOT TOLERATE DEEP SUCTIONING. IT MAKES ME WORSE. PLEASE PUSH ON MY STOMACH INSTEAD. THIS CLEARS MY LUNGS MORE EFFECTIVELY.

Twenty years later, in 1997, I was having some persistent breathing problems which were different from anything I had ever experienced before. I kept going to my pulmonologist and he kept writing me prescriptions, but nothing seemed to help. Also, although I had not noticed it, I had basically stopped eating. For many years it had been difficult for me to swallow, and I spent an average of four hours a day trying to force food into my body. Gradually, I ate less and less until I was consuming just a few bites each day. Finally, I checked myself into a local hospital.

Things went downhill quickly. In retrospect, there were three factors which contributed to the disaster that followed. The first was that members of the hospital staff brought their own set of assumptions about me. If I had not been so sick, I could have engaged them in interesting conversations about my life and work. I had done this in previous hospitalizations and had better interactions with the staff. The second problem, related to the first, was that people did not listen to me. I brought thirty-five years of experience with my body, and while it was true that I needed their knowledge and expertise, they also needed mine. Third, I was used to counting on my circle in many areas of my life, but I tended to keep friends at a distance whenever I was in the hospital. It was mostly vanity and a reluctance to inconvenience people. I found it impossible to have a good visit amid the interruptions and chaos of a busy hospital floor, and I wanted to be attentive to my guests. If I couldn't do that, I didn't want any guests. Ultimately, it was this mistake that nearly cost me my life.

Misunderstandings about who I was began the moment I was admitted. While I was being transferred from the emergency room stretcher to my hospital bed, the nursing assistant asked, "What house are you from?" From the way she phrased the question, I knew she was asking which group home I lived in. I said, "I have my own home in Manchester." Whether this had any impact, I do not know. She did not ask me anything else.

Shortly thereafter, a nurse came in with a clipboard and asked me a lot of admitting questions. In addition to my medical history and allergies, she wanted detailed information about where I lived, where I worked, what I did about transportation, how I was supported in my home, and so on. I was pleased that she seemed interested in capturing the entire picture of my life.

Unfortunately, neither this nurse nor any of the other staff seemed to absorb any of my responses. For most of my time in the hospital, I overheard people talking about me. They made up stories about where I had come from and how I lived, but I was too weak to correct them. Even more frightening, I eventually lost my connection with who I had been. I knew the stories were wrong, but I could not remember enough about my life to convince even myself that I had been so capable at one time.

The one beautiful exception to the low expectations surrounding me was an APRN (Assistant Physician/Registered Nurse). My mother had previously taken a class from her, and when they reunited on my hospital floor and my mother introduced us, we were all so happy to be together. My circle quickly named her the Good Nurse. She had a background in rehabilitation, and understood immediately the importance of getting me home to my life and normal activities. Throughout the rest of my stay, she served as my advocate and adviser, and sometimes as my co-conspirator. The Good Nurse and my circle are two of the main reasons I survived this experience.

On the morning of the third day, I dictated a message to my mother so she could give it to the doctor when he came by later in the afternoon. It read: "Please help me. I am too tired to breathe or to eat. Please put a tube up my nose to feed me, and put a bipap on to breathe for me. I can't go on like this anymore." A bipap is an external ventilator which blows air into the nose through a mask. It is a non-invasive device I had seen in a magazine a few weeks before. I had always had a pretty good relationship with this doctor. He listened to me and apparently trusted my judgement. We seemed to be off to a good start again, and he signed the orders to carry out my requests. Soon after, people came in and started packing up my belongings. I was being moved to intensive care.

Suddenly, I was terrified. Were they going to use a bipap, or were they going to use the more traditional trach? I had been avoiding a tracheostomy ever since that pneumonia so long ago. A trach had always been the quick answer whenever people didn't know what else to do about my breathing problems. But I could not bear the thought of living without my voice. My body is so fragile. Whenever someone is moving me, I give constant verbal instructions so that I do not sprain muscles or break bones.

I started asking frantic questions about what was going to happen next. I wanted promises that I would not lose my voice or have a trach put in against my will. I must have asked too many questions because a nurse approached with a syringe and injected the liquid (Atavan) into my intravenous line. She was speaking gently, saying that I was getting myself all upset, and that this would help me to relax.

UPSET? OF COURSE I WAS UPSET! People were not answering my questions or speaking with me as if I had any choice about what was done to my body. My concerns about being heard grew larger and larger. The Atavan was continued every few hours, and was supplemented by sleeping pills and other calming agents.

A good moment in my hospital visit was when Dr. Russman came to see me. He was an international expert about my disability, and I had been a patient of his for many years. The hospital had invited his input about my eating problem. When Dr. Russman suggested that I have a G-tube (gastric tube) put in, I was overjoyed. One of my unstated dreams was to not have to struggle with eating anymore. The doctor described how a G-tube works, and even said that if I wanted to eat by mouth I could still do that.

Of course, knowing what needs to be done and getting it done are two different things. I endured several more days of having a feeding tube up my nose before I could be scheduled for the G-tube procedure. There are three ways to put in a G-tube. The safest and most common way is to go down the person's throat, but my disability has changed the shape of my mouth and throat so much that I knew this would be impossible. I am only able to open my mouth a little bit, and my head remains in a fixed position toward the right. If someone tries to open my mouth any farther or turns my head to midline, my throat closes and I cannot breathe. I explained this at great length to a number of people.

On Thursday morning, I arrived in the procedure room and was told they would be going down my throat. We went back and forth and I agreed to let them try. When I woke up, I was told "We could not get the tube in. Every time we tried to move your head, your oxygen level would go down." I'm not sure whether I said "I told you so," but they knew. The trouble was that they wouldn't remember the next time.

Later that day I was scheduled to have the G-tube put in the second way, in the radiology lab. This went better at first, but by evening I was in incredible pain. The next day nurses hung bags of food from IV polls and it trickled into my stomach through a long tube. The pain gradually subsided but was replaced by bloating. I told the nurse I was being fed too much. When the bloating continued and grew worse, I complained more frequently and was given suppositories.

By Saturday I was in agony. Of course, my mother was there every day, and over the weekend several friends stopped by to see me. Everybody exclaimed that I looked pregnant. The hospital staff did not seem to think this was unusual, so we just waited for the bloating to go down.

Late Monday afternoon, the Good Nurse came by with a rectal tube to try to relieve some of the pressure. My friend Sarah was there, and they tried rolling me from side to side in search of some relief. Next, the Good Nurse tried draining some of the food out of my stomach through the G-tube in case I was actually being fed too much. Nothing worked.

Tuesday the Good Nurse pressed on my abdomen and looked concerned. "You are as hard as a drum," she said, and sent me immediately for x-rays. It turned out that air was leaking out of my digestive tract and being trapped inside my belly. The Good Nurse and several doctors met me back at my hospital room and told me I was going for emergency surgery. Until now, I had been anesthetized with "twilight" medications which do not require breathing support. This time I was going under general anesthetic and would have to be on a ventilator (the traditional kind that I feared so much). All of us were concerned about whether I would ever be able to come off the ventilator, but there was no choice.

I was also worried that because of the structure of my throat, it might be impossible to intubate me without doing a tracheostomy. I begged them to find another way, and learned that the tube could be put up my nose instead. Although the process was awful (I had to be awake to help them find my trachea), I was glad to find this new option. I was also happy because the hospital people were finally saying, "We need you to help us with this." Once again, it might have meant an ongoing change in how I was treated, but it faded away as soon as the crisis was over.

I spoke briefly with my mother over the phone, and I had tearful but optimistic words with Stephen and with my friend Kathy who happened to be visiting when this all happened. Then I was whisked off to surgery. As I rolled down the hall on a stretcher, watching the ceiling lights pass by, I kept thanking God for my life, my parents, my friends, and all the opportunities that had come my way. I wanted more years, but I would never have traded the years I had already experienced.

The surgery went extremely well and when I awoke, still on the ventilator, the pain and bloating were gone. I had a sprained knee, probably from being catheterized, but it was not terribly painful and it could have been so much worse. I decided that I needed to go home. But there were still a few hurdles to get over first.

I had originally gone into the hospital because I felt like I could not breathe. Except when people were doing weird things to my neck, the oxygen sensor on my finger never showed alarmingly low levels. Still, it felt like something was wrong with my breathing. Requests for assisted coughing brought responses like "We don't do that here. The liability is too great. We might rupture your liver. Would you like to be suctioned?" Of course, I always refused. I knew the consequences. But as time went on and no progress was made toward helping me breathe more easily, I became increasingly desperate.

One day, when the doctor came through on rounds, I begged him to do something about my breathing. A respiratory therapist was standing near me. She had been doing breathing treatments with me throughout my hospital stay, and I liked her. The doctor looked in her direction and said, "Suction her." I knew in that moment that he didn't know how to help me and was giving up. I don't know why I didn't fight. Maybe the Atavan had made me too mellow for my own good. I thought, "I haven't been suctioned in twenty years. What could be the harm in trying it just this once?" Besides, I trusted this therapist. She was friendly and wanted to help me. So I let her try. My intensive care nurse was there too.

The therapist inserted the tube into my nose, but once again, the peculiar shape of my neck was an obstacle. The tube kept coming out through my mouth. That was the good news. The bad news was that with persistence, she was eventually able to get the tube into my lungs. I began to die. The fear was gone and I laid there passively while the nurse said, "She's starting to de-sat" (meaning my oxygen level was dropping)! The respiratory therapist quickly withdrew the tube, and the two of them spoke back and forth in serious tones. They looked really worried.

In desperation, the nurse began to press on my stomach, trying to produce an assisted cough. But this technique doesn't work unless I participate and cough in unison with the other person. I just watched the whole scene, with interest but without emotion. For a time, I literally did not care if I never took another breath. Then, gradually, I began to cough and to return to life. After that, I had better luck getting people to cough with me.

With all these experiences, it became clear to my circle that the best thing to do was to get me out of there. I was not only in real physical danger, but was quickly sinking into despair as well.

My friend Faith suggested that the circle keep a journal beside my hospital bed, and that everyone write something in it during each visit. Topics included my stated issues and concerns, conversations with medical staff, and things the staff said to or about me. Here are some excerpts from this journal. No wonder I was losing heart.

◆ Peggy (Cathy's mom) – We are concerned about doing assisted coughing (pushing on Cathy's stomach) with a G-tube. Will this be possible? The doctor says she would need to be trached first.

◆ Cathy – I breathe better lying down, but tube feedings have to be done sitting up. If I sit up, I can't breathe; if I lie down, I can't eat!

◆ Unsigned – Speaking of moving ahead, how can Cathy get her life back with all these new fangled gadgets and life changes? We're worried a bit that people around her now are seeing her as fragile rather than focusing on her tremendous capacity as an independent woman.

◆ Peggy – I asked the nurse (Barbara) about bolus feeding, and she said the same thing Cathy has been hearing – that the hospital does not do this because people cannot absorb the proper nutrients unless the food is dripped in slowly

◆ Sarah to [the Good Nurse] – Would you consider adding in the chart a request that people not make indiscriminate comments about Cathy needing a trach, not being able to live independently, etc.?

The circle set up a schedule of visitors so that people would be with me during most of each day. They reached out to my wider group of friends, coworkers, spouses of friends and coworkers, and community people, and told all of them I needed to be protected and supported.

The circle held a meeting at my home to hash out issues and create an escape plan. The Good Nurse was consulted and brought into the process as a key player. She advised me to tell the nursing staff that when I returned home I was going to be bolus feeding (consuming an entire can of G-tube food all at once), and that the doctor wanted the nurses to teach me how this was done so that I could teach my support staff. I was to punctuate this request with little anecdotes about taking my lunch to work, going out with friends, and other normal activities where I did not want to be toting an IV pole around with me.

This turned the tide. I did not feel confident, but I hid under this fictitious doctor's order and the nurses all went along. They even allowed me to instruct them about doing a bolus feeding because I wanted the practice.

We got me home. The only new thing being done for my lungs was a prescription for Claritin to reduce my allergies. But I seemed to be breathing better, and at this point I was making brave statements about preferring to die at home should it come to that. When I rolled into my living room and looked around, however, I knew something was really wrong. Nothing looked familiar at all. I could not remember how to schedule staff. I no longer knew how to coach people through the delicate process of moving me. I barely knew my own name. We referred to the hospital journal and noticed that over 22 days I had been given Heparin, Atavan, Resteral, Xanax, Albuterol, Cromolyn, Claritin, Theophylline, Prednisone, twilight anesthetic, general anesthetic, and post-op pain medication.

I absolutely could not function, and in some ways this was more frightening than being unable to breathe. Most of my circle (about 10 people) accompanied me back to the emergency room. The hospital was not sure what to do with so many visitors, but my friends had all decided that I would not be left alone with strangers. I was admitted to a psychiatric hospital for a few days, and members of my circle stayed with me day and night. Free of all medications, my thinking became clearer, and I was soon ready to go home and start the next stage of my life.

My first concern was to reconnect with all the people who didn't know what had happened to me. I had piles of mail and dozens of phone messages from friends and associates, and the idea of getting back to everyone was overwhelming. So I wrote a letter, a pretty frank letter, about surviving the hospital. I also sent the letter to members of my circle, and to other people who had shared the experience. My friend Julie responded with this email:

Dear Cathy,

Your email came through just fine. Having just talked with you in the afternoon, I was full of awareness of all that you did not say in your letter. What you wrote was beautifully concise and expressive - and appropriate to the venue. And what you experienced during that month was so complex and significant for you that you couldn't put it into "update" format anyway, I'm sure. I admire and respect your willingness to struggle with the complexity, your commitment to discover the meaning and significance, and I am deeply appreciative of your willingness to share that exploration with me. It would be easy to say "I was sick and now I'm better" or "it was the medication," because those are true statements. The path you have chosen takes courage, but can bring you to such wonderful and unexpected places. I am reminded, as Aeschylus phrased it, that there are times when "... pain falls drop by drop upon the heart. [But] in our own despair, against our will, comes wisdom, through the awful grace of God."

Julie

A couple of months later, I had a party to celebrate my escape from the hospital. I put out snacks, along with plastic knives, forks, spoons, and bolus syringes! I bought gold and white balloons, tied them in bunches onto cans of Jevity (G-tube food), and scattered them throughout the house. I made two big blue display boards full of affirmations, thankful thoughts, and pictures of Stephen and me in Newport, Rhode Island (so much for hospital predictions that I could never go anywhere now that I had a G-tube).

I also wrote something to put on the display board. When I was in the hospital and too weak to keep explaining to everyone about my life, I kept overhearing staff members as they discussed my case and my life. There was an alarming amount of misinformation, and it almost seemed as if they had created another person and placed her in my body. As a way to release some of my anger about this, and as an educational tool, I wrote a short piece. Then I thought, "I was pretty heavily medicated… Maybe I should run this by somebody before I go public with it." So I sent it to the Good Nurse. Later I called her and asked if I had accurately portrayed the staff's comments about me. Her response was simple but chilling: "You were so kind to them."

Then the Good Nurse asked me to print the piece in the largest type I could fit on one sheet of paper, and plastered it up all over the hospital.

Here is what I wrote…

PERCEPTIONS . . .

The Assumption

She has spent all her life in institutions. Never read a book or wrote a letter. Never went to a movie. Never had a job. The nursing home sent her here because she got sick. We'll do our best to patch her up because we believe that every life is important, no matter how miserable. If she recovers, we'll send her back to the nursing home, where she'll live out the rest of her useless days. Then she'll die.

The Truth

She grew up in a family that loved her. Her parents thought of her as having much potential. College was always assumed, and she graduated with honors. Now nationally recognized, she writes books and articles, counsels individuals and groups, and travels over a large area to share her knowledge. Always popular, she surrounds herself with wonderful people whose commitment sustains her through the hard times. She lives on her own, in a home that belongs to her. She plans to get married. Life is good.

When a person cannot speak for herself,
the assumption pulsates loudly,
while the truth only whispers.

Care enough to learn the truth.
Then dare to pass it on!

When we met Regina, she was living in a nursing facility. Through her efforts and those of her circle of support, she was able to move into the community. First she moved into the home of friends, later into her own apartment, and now she owns her own home. A talented writer and professional counselor, Regina has much to offer to society. She was startled, however, by the reversal of roles when she assumed responsibility for her mother in her final months.

MOTHER AND CHILD REUNION
Regina DeMarassé

"But Regina, your mother has to have a primary caregiver to remain with us in the Visiting Nurse Association, and you're it."

Transportation was the issue. Only months before, the Amyotrophic Lateral Sclerosis (ALS) Association had video-taped my mother leaving her home in Queens to take the subway to the ALS Center in Manhattan. ALS (Lou Gerig's Disease) is a motor-neuron condition in which movement of nearly all skeletal muscles is slowly lost, due to nerve death. Mom was still quite ambulatory. The association called the video *Living with ALS*. Now that Mom was living with me in Connecticut, however, eight decades of subway travel meant nothing.

My concern was Mom didn't know her way around Waterbury. Her doctors and their offices were all new. She could barely hold up her head to look around. Should she get lost, she had no voice to speak. She had long since given up trying to get strangers to understand her circumstances.

At first, people shied away from Mom when the difficulty in her speech became more pronounced. Cards she carried explained her condition, but I'm not sure if she ever used them. Writing notes to continue one's communications as one travels about is not too expeditious, especially in winter. It becomes particularly ridiculous when, instead of speaking, people start responding with notes.

All I wanted was an escort to accompany Mom door-to-door to her appointments. I am blind.

It was two years before, when Mom was reading me questions from my National Certified Counsel review book, that I first noticed the slur. Already counseling clients at a generic agency, I needed to pass my comprehensives and later the boards, if there was to be a life after internship. I was desperate to find enough readers to help me prepare. Mom was visiting and bailed me out.

The slur was initially diagnosed as resulting from a mini-stroke. The degree of speech impairment continued to progress, however. Two days after my grad school commencement, ALS was diagnosed. I am forever grateful it wasn't diagnosed two days before I graduated (with honors), besmirching one of the proudest days in Mom's life.

Labels have always existed. Because she was female, my mother wasn't afforded the same opportunities her brothers were. Mom wasn't given the opportunity to attend college. She felt no shame in washing other people's toilets to make ends meet, but she still would have loved the chance to continue her education. Mom was determined to see her four children get that chance.

They did. For me it took thirteen years to acquire my first degree, after a benign upper spinal tumor left me blind and quadriplegic. With the determination given me through my immigrant grandmother to my mother, I did it. Family and friends helped, as did social service agencies, college personnel and fellow students. I didn't, however, attend that graduation, feeling out of sinc with my peers.

It wasn't until I heard the mourn in my mother's voice over possibly missing my second graduation, that I decided to change plans and attend it. Sherri, my assistant, offered to rise at 4:30 a.m. to do what it takes to get someone else's motionless body washed, dressed, fed, and halfway across the state in time for a 9:00 assembly and a 10:00 processional. Seven years later, Dave did the same for a downstate trek.

Some weeks after the downstate trek, Dave, my friend and live-in assistant of several years, heard Mom's diagnosis, after it was confirmed beyond a doubt. "She should come live with us," were his next words. "Getting an aide for a longer shift to do two people is often easier than finding someone for one." Since Dave was my sole backup caregiver and maintenance man, this would be quite a bit of responsibility for him to take on. The in-law apartment Mom would occupy had originally been intended for *his* backup support. I was going to give him two weeks to reconsider.

Many years it had been my heart's desire to look after my mother in her old age. Through all my days and long nights of pain, when the tumor had been actively hammering away at my nervous system, Mom had been there. Her faith for me and in me had been relentless. Her devotion was unsurpassed. With her help, I beat the odds of a terminal disease. The tumor ceased. Paralysis didn't.

One doesn't come away from a situation like that mildly affected. Both caregiver and care-receiver are forever changed. When the two are so close they share the experience as one, as did Mom and I, the difference between giver and receiver begins melding. It is only bodies that separate us.

Dave got one week. Taking on responsibility for Mom's care was not her payback, it was my need. It was a precious opportunity to experience an ever-deepening fount of love - one that in his later care for Mom, Dave also felt.

"Oh no, no. You can't do that," was the general reaction to my proposal - a blind and quadriplegic daughter - to look after the affairs of an ever-failing mother. Then when they considered how with team support of family and friends I had left an institution, finished college, got a career, got a house of my own, they reconsidered. After all, who else in the family had a network of aides already at hand? Who else was as well-equipped to hire and train than Dave and Regina? Who else already knew how to plod through the quicksand of bureaucracy? And who else considered, in depth, the emotional and physical challenges of sitting inside a body first in rebellion, later in desertion.

As Mom's speech became more and more garbled, her swallowing came less and less. Paralysis was slowly creeping down her body. Just about everything affected on Mom was not affected on me. Initially, just about everything affected on me, was not affected on Mom, at least not in the same way.

Since my sighted and able-bodied days working at The Mayor's Office for the Handicapped in New York City, I feared encounters with non-fluent speakers. It wasn't that I lacked patience or felt put-off. It wasn't that I determined them imbecilic or too sick to be worthy of my attention. I lacked confidence. Believing myself to be a kind and loving person, I somehow felt I should be able to listen with *perfect* understanding to all persons. When I didn't succeed, I didn't want to face my inability. I didn't want to be part of that person's frustration.

Some years later, blindness further compromised such communications, with the elimination of facial cues. At the rehab center, I wised-up; I listened that much more intently to non-fluent people. When I didn't understand, we simply tried again. It occurred to me it was cruel to avoid a fellow human being simply out of fear.

Just before Mom conceded to typing her communications into a small computer that spoke, she told my sister-in-law, "Regina understands me the best."

Rounding-up enough help for Mom and me was not always easy, but one way or another, it happened. There were some good days we had together, and some I wouldn't want to revisit. I was honored that Mom chose to spend her final days with me. It would have been wonderful if Mom's health held out 'til Spring so she could see the beautiful gardens David had planted beyond her back door, but I suppose we always want more time. There is always more beauty to hear, to see, to feel, and more love to share. Our Creator has given abundantly.

Until the last months of Mom's life, we maintained hope for a healing. We did not want her to meet her death with tremendous suffering. In the end, my prayers were answered. The ALS took lungs before limbs, saving Mom the frustration of not only being unable to move, but not having a voice to even ask for help blowing her nose.

Life in the body must end, and Mom's had been a long one, mostly in good health. Since she was eight years old and had a little brother, she had often been a caregiver: for four children, for her mother, for her husband, and for me. Seldom had anyone, besides perhaps my father, nurtured her... not even her own detached mother.

People loved caring for my mom. She not only needed assistance with tasks of daily living, but also hot packs and massage, patience and concern. With my aides and my friends – not put off by a failing body – Mom finally had to accept the fussing and support she had long since deserved. I believe Mom received a healing to her soul.

So I have been a caregiver.

HONEST, I DIDN'T RAIN ON THEIR PARADE

Regina DeMarassé

The day after Mom's service - the service with the perfect weather - it rained for two weeks. One of those very rainy days, May 23rd, was the second anniversary of my grad school commencement. It had rained that day too, all over the football field through which my wheelchair was supposed to roll up to the stage. We counselors (human service workers) always get the short shaft, like being way, way back. Behind us were the beaming mommies and daddies.

Anyway, the Jesuits were not pleased with my insistence to sit at the back of the field. They thought I'd slow down the procession. My classmates and I were relentless that I belonged with my class, and that they were perfectly capable of pushing me up to the front.

The rain commenced as did the 9:00 a.m. train of girls, boys, women and men with black squares on their heads. (I was already seated.). It wasn't too chilly, not yet. By the time all the heart titillating, sage, and angel-winged pronouncements were done, a decision was made to skip the trot to the podium and go home.

Honest, it wasn't me. I don't make the weather. Apparently, the Jesuits in their concerns about perfect processions hadn't checked-in with He who does.

Anyhow, this year the winds also howled on May 23rd. I remembered graduation and put on beads of Mom's that had been given to me at her service. Although the day was cold, damp and dreary, as her beads touched the back of my neck, they had not the slightest chill.

I close this section with a story I wrote about my mother, who passed away the week before Mother's Day in 1998. Although this is about her death, it is also about her life and her lasting influence on me.

NOT ALONE IN THE WORLD
Cathy Ludlum

It was one of those midnight phone calls that you hope you will never get, but we all seem to get eventually.

"This is Officer C. from the Wethersfield Police Department. We are trying to locate a relative of Peggy Ludlum. Are you her sister?"

"No, I am her daughter," I said, suddenly wide awake. "What's happened?"

"She called 911, and the ambulance has transported her to the hospital."

"How is she?"

"I'm sorry to have to tell you this, but she wasn't doing very well when they took her out of here."

I was miles away. I was in Maryland at my first national business meeting since my serious illness the previous year. Mom had been extremely worried about me getting sick on the trip, and I kept saying I would be fine. I had a G-tube now, and I was healthier than I had been in years. Maybe she had a premonition that something big was going to happen while I was gone... but this was the last thing I expected.

Other than calling the emergency room and speaking with the doctor in charge (who was also not saying anything encouraging), there wasn't anything I could do right then. So I told my assistant to go back to sleep and I laid awake planning and remembering.

My father died when I was eight years old. It seemed as though all of my life I had feared losing my mother and being all alone in the world. There were many times it looked as if I would go first, but my mother never accepted that idea. She believed I would have a happy and long life. She worked hard to prepare the way for me by making sure my educational, social, and medical needs were met. She also prepared me to take advantage of all the opportunities she believed would be coming my way.

Early in the morning, I was on the phone making arrangements. I called the director of my agency, who was at the same Maryland conference. She immediately relieved me of any further responsibilities and told me to go home. When I had spoken to the hospital in the middle of the night, the nurse kept asking me for relatives close-by in Connecticut. She had said something about needing to make decisions… So I called Bernie, a doctor and close family friend, and my circle member Faith who had been such a great advocate during my own hospital stay. I explained the situation to them, and said, "I am asking you to act as family until I can get home." And of course they said yes. I called my roommate to tell her I was coming back early and asked her to relay the news to my other personal assistants. I had some things to wrap up at the hotel, and then we loaded my van and started the long drive home.

We did not know in the beginning that the key to my independence would be interdependence: the ability to engage people in my life while offering them my particular gifts and talents. It has always been easy for me to make friends. It is both a joy and a survival strategy. When my circle of support began, it was a wonderful revelation to find that people besides my mother were committed to my well-being. As I gained more autonomy through the support of my friends, and later my personal assistants, my mother struggled with feelings of protectiveness. It would have been easy for her to put up roadblocks. But she knew the best thing she could do would be to allow me to reduce my dependence upon her.

By the time we got home, nine hours later, it was dark out and I was in no shape to go to the hospital. I kept in phone contact with the nurse, and she reported that my mother was still unresponsive. Faith and Bernie had each been there, and each had conversations with the doctors and nurses caring for my mom. We were all trying to find something hopeful in this situation, but we were not having much success. My mother had been living with emphysema for many years. Maintaining her breathing had come to require many breathing treatments, medications, and inhalers used at various times during the day. Even so, she had remained active, carrying a portable nebulizer around in her car. This turn of events was not all that surprising. Even so, none of us wanted to let her go.

It takes a strong person to let a child with a disability take the risks that are necessary to having a full life. In agreeing with my move into the co-op, my mother made it possible for me to create a stable support system which could endure for decades. It was hard for her to reduce her physical support of me. Almost until the last month of her life, she was still asking me if I needed her to help me in the bathroom, even though we had not done this together for over five years. But she continued to watch out for me, bringing me clippings about fire safety, and always providing a listening ear when I needed to figure out something in my life.

It was a strange thing to go into the intensive care unit to see my mother. We had played this scene out so many times, but I had always been the patient. This time she was relying on me to make the necessary decisions. I was a bit overwhelmed by the responsibility. She looked so small lying there with all those tubes. Faith placed my hand on my mother's, and I tried to talk to her, but my voice kept breaking. The ventilator made its rhythmic sound. There were lots of tests to determine the level of brain damage my mother had undergone during her most recent breathing episode. It was a long week of waiting and worrying and wondering what to do next. A number of people from my circle came by to see her. We decorated her room in her favorite color by bringing red cards and red balloons. The whole time, my mother's words kept echoing in my head: "If something happens to me, and I will be permanently unconscious and kept alive only by tubes, that is not what I want." Organized to the last, my mother had prepared a Living Will which expressed her wishes in more detail.

Abraham Lincoln said, "All that I am, I owe to my mother." My mom did many things to help me become an independent, creative, determined, and resilient adult. But the best thing she ever did was to give me the skills and the opportunities I needed to form strong and lasting friendships. Her passing was a devastating loss. But because of her, I will never be alone in the world.

DON'T FORGET TO HAVE FUN

Everyone has a lot to do. People with disabilities, elders, and their families and friends have even more to keep track of and worry about. If it isn't a problem with supports, it is a problem with equipment. If it isn't that, it is setting up a half-dozen meetings as part of pursuing a goal. It's easy to get caught up in survival issues and to minimize the importance of social and recreational activities.

But today is the only day we have. Let's enjoy it!

Learning to Play

Having fun *does* not have to be complicated or expensive. Although taking a vacation to a far-away place is great once in awhile, there are little things we can do right now to break the patterns of stress and repetition.

- ♦ Start a video night
- ♦ Go to the park
- ♦ Call an old friend that you haven't talked to in a long time
- ♦ Sleep late
- ♦ Attend a town festival
- ♦ Cook something new
- ♦ Work in the garden
- ♦ Talk with a neighbor
- ♦ Watch the sun come up or go down
- ♦ Have a party!

One day I was feeling particularly upset, and wrote down a bunch of things that make me happy. If you like that idea, you can make your own list. The challenging part is to actually DO some of those things. Start small, and make a game out of it. And remember, many of these activities are more fun when shared with a friend!

Things That Make Me Happy

All music, but especially
    Soothing music
    Music from Ireland and Scotland
    Instrumental jazz
    Opera
Flowers (in manageable amounts)
Being out with friends
Going places
Doing things
Restaurants
Movies – especially classics
Concerts
Plays
Poetry readings
Talks
Parties
Small gatherings where I can hear and be heard
Rollerskating (or other large spaces where I can drive FAST)
Meeting new people
Talking with friends on the phone
Getting things done
Cleaning
Order (vs. disorder)
Seeing a difference
Knowing where things are
Knowing when things are
Being surrounded with kindred spirits
Being listened to
Dreaming
Helping other people reach their dreams
Writing something good
Giving a good talk
Facilitating a good meeting
Making a difference
Playing Scrabble (without scoring)
Doing computer things with people (especially people who know more about computers than I do)
Experimenting with clothes/different looks, etc.
Shocking people (as in "You did WHAT?!?)
My G-tube
Being warm, but not hot
A gentle rain
A downpour (if I'm inside)
A sunrise
A sunset
A beautiful blue sky
Looking at the stars
Praying , when I'm "into it"
Saying no
Remembering my mom
Remembering my dad
Songs/articles/artifacts from their generation (1940's and 1950's)
Family
Being able to cry when I need to
Balance
Not too much of anything, including all of the above

Things That DON'T Make Me Happy

Country-Western music
Surprises
Feeling trapped
Being in places that are too loud or too crowded
Not knowing what to do (about some situation)
Having too much to do

Of course, there is nothing better than getting away and leaving the problems at home. Although travel creates its own type of stress, the benefits of being in a different place with different people can be enormous. If the opportunity arises, don't be afraid to enjoy new experiences and make new memories.

ACROSS THE POND
Regina DeMarasse

In the spring of 2002, the Circles Network (in England) invited Communitas (in New England) to return for another series of conferences. Ten of us took off from Boston on September 12th to share our visions and experiences of inclusion of people with disabilities in community.

I can hardly believe these Brits asked me back a second time. They paid accommodations just to hear my babble, along with what my more engaging colleagues had to say. The Brits seem to appreciate our pioneering spirit.

We were a team of eight adults and two teens, ambulatory and not so ambulatory, with and without labels - and I don't mean clothing tags. It would take many pages to describe how each person added to the bouquet. So I shall be superficial - mostly - and focus on my own adventure.

Despite my body's grumblings, I certainly had a wonderful week. There was incredible team support from both sides. There also had to be tremendous work behind the scenes. We had a number of blunders in timing, as a big group is bound to have, but people kept pulling together to work things out. Humor came later.

The first conference was in London, at the Cricket Grounds. Through a miscommunication we wound up taking the first black cabby that stopped: a rickety old thing. I just rolled in (no lock-downs) as I had done in the previous cab, but that was a younger, smoother, version. Then I bounced and veered with every bump. I thought I would die.

Anyway, the first conference was on children, and I'm afraid our first two days for me has blended into a London fog. (By the way, the true weather the whole week was rather lovely)

Some of us decided to leave early the next day for the country. When we switched on the radio in our room at the inn near Rugby, the tune was from Cabaret: "Welcome" in half a dozen languages. Things would be getting better.

At the second conference, a video was shown after lunch. The Irish fellow narrating told of a life of physical limitation that opened up with the help of a person-centered plan and a circle of support. Hearing elements of my own story told in a brogue was quite a surprise. It went straight to my heart.

Bringing one's immediate community together in a circle of support, as we do it these days, began with a Canadian. Judith Snow was fighting for her life and to have a life. She was exhausted. Her friends needed her, and broke ground to help her find a way out of an institution.

The concept of circles of support traveled to Connecticut and other states and provinces. Then a few North Americans brought it across the ocean to open lives for the diverse members of the United Kingdom.

Speaking of circles, was it the next day we visited Avery? Such is a site of some pretty big rocks. The whole town is within parts of a circle in which these seven (or was it twelve?) stones stand. They are not piled, as at Stonehenge, but they are not fenced off either. George, a former seminarian, touched one for me and then touched me. I said a prayer.

Maybe that's why my life is changing.

Two days later, we moved on to the conference in Somerset. This was my big moment to deliver an address on "The Price of Freedom," during which twice my throat went dry. Fortunately, Pat had my cheat sheet and filled in while I was administered water and eucalyptus lozenges.

For me, the highlight that day came when my old buddy Phil the Brit showed up, taking some time from his UPS rep job to deliver hugs, kisses, and a warm exchange. An entire decade melted away. The grapevine had taken care to see Phil was informed that I was back on his side of the pond. And no one seemed to mind that I played hookey from the group session after lunch.

The finale of this conference was singing along to a tune by James Keelaghan:

>...Well the ride is never free
>Always gonna be a price to pay
>But I can tell you that it's worth the ticket
>If you want to see a brighter day

Never gonna stop this train
Never gonna stop this train
It left the station a long time ago
Never gonna stop this train

James is probably not aware he is now the author of a dance tune. Brits and Yanks got up and formed a conga line. Pretty soon even I hitched on.

No one is ever going to stop this train.

In one week, we not only hit 3 locales for 3 conferences, where we gave spiels of different lengths and then collaborated with others, but we got to play!

The next day was Stratford on Avon. Geese, swans and ducks were also on Avon, having a lot to say about how us touristy types should feed them. Oliver Twist they were not.

We did such grand things as buying socks and ties that had Shakespearian quotes along with books on English gardens, and just enjoyed a bit of sunshine while starlings sang about I know not what.

Word came that Evensong was to be heard at Coventry Cathedral. Mandy shot off all over Stratford, in a heroic effort to round up the rest of the team to convene a half hour early for the performance. Miraculously, at her very last stop, she found the Hood family in a second floor tea room…

The organ was fabulous, the girls' choir sweet. Eventually, we were politely kicked out by a deacon or something, after the young fellow at the organ unleashed a most magnificent chord progression that seemed to fill all living space. An advantage to being blind and lacking other sensory perception is, in such places and in such moments, my whole world is just music. Ommm.

Ruins of a 14th century cathedral were apparent through a glass wall. The old cathedral was partially destroyed during the war. The new one was built or completed in 1962, after 20 years of planning. Coventry being a laborers' town, Jesus is depicted in a carpenter's apron. The tradition of the 75 years of work it took to build the original structure was carried on by the sweat of these workers, resurrecting their cathedral.

Triumphing over bombs that 20th century day of sirens, horror, and screams, the steeple of the old structure remains, ever reaching upwards more than 900 feet. Within the new cathedral, tapestries and other gifts from the Germans ask forgiveness. I wish it all could serve as a reminder. Heaven help us.

In the last year, much of my life and my dreams also seemed in ruins. Despite being unsettled at home, I resurrected to the invite to England. Purpose has returned, the fruits of my labors.

The new cathedral, by the way, lacks the impressive steps of the old. That's cool. It's wheelchair accessible!

Back on pavement after supper in a pub, a cascade of bells resounded left, right, from all around us. Every fifteen minutes, this celebration pealed forth. Actually, it all came from one moderately sized "Trinity Church" nearby, but such is the quality of non-electric chimes: they fill even the ethers. Was this grand display for us? (I don't think so.)

Throughout the week, we were wined and dined repeatedly, gratifying both my interests in exotic food and down home English favorites. Good conversation also was included.

Unplanned were the birds, big and small, that pleased and amused me with their vocalizations in the Midlands, Stratford, and Bourton on the Water.

The eighth morning, we packed up to return to London, then home, arriving there 19 hours later.

The week had been far more active (physically) than most for me, but getting through proved I'm still young. Actually, with a few more early nights and a slight increase in rest periods, I could have gone another week or two. The plane ride home, however, left me achy, then quiet and unproductive my first days back. Eight hours for my body in those quaint seats can do that. So can jet lag, I suppose.

Then after three days, I made a remarkable recovery and had a surge of energy. In spirit, the trip renewed me. Britain was just a lovely thing to do at this particular time in my life. It was actually salvation.

Now it is back to business - you know, the price of freedom.

One Candle Power is about recognizing gifts, your own as well as those of the people around you, and how these gifts might best be used for the benefit of others. So often, these gifts become apparent when people gather to share food, music, and conversation. People who arrive lonely or tired leave feeling accepted and energized. From baby showers to Sweet Sixteens, from weddings to retirement parties, the momentous occasions of our lives are a reason to bring people together. It is about something more than the event itself; it is about relationships and community.

What better way to end this exploration of One Candle Power than with a celebration?

LIFE IS A GIFT
Cathy Ludlum

As much as my life has been full of friendship, laughter, fun, and adventure; it has been equally full of situations that might have meant my demise. I have experienced bad medical decisions and close calls in my van. I have slipped underwater in swimming pools and bathtubs, and had pneumonias which were like drowning on dry land. Fortunately, someone has always been there to pull me out of the water or push on my stomach to help me cough. But it is impossible for me to go very long without recognizing the little miracles which allow each of us to live another day.

So when I was about 38, I started planning a GIANT 40th birthday celebration. I picked a date and started thinking about what I wanted to have happen. Yes, I wanted a big party, but I wanted it to be more than that. I have relationships that go back for decades, and I have new friends who are an important part of my life now. There are also people who know me less well, but we are connected professionally, and I hoped to show my appreciation for their support. In addition, I had a desire for pomp and circumstance similar to a wedding, but didn't necessarily want to get married. When I heard about how Gunner Dybwad (a renowned advocate in the field of mental retardation) held a "90th birthday conference," my ideas began to take a more definite form.

The party continued to simmer in the background for another year. Then in the summer of 2001, I gave it a name, "Life Is a Gift." My circle and

I went to work as if we were planning a small conference. Friends helped research locations while I talked to kosher caterers. Some aspects of the event were already determined because I wanted to adhere to traditional Jewish practices, but there was lots of room for innovation as well. A circle member designed and printed the invitations, and we had several small gatherings to address them (about 200 envelopes). I made silly nametags, and dug out copies of books I had written so we could put them on display.

The preparations were arduous and time-consuming, but amazing things were happening even then. I asked my close friend Janice if she would sing, and almost immediately her son, a musician, said he wanted to write a song for the occasion. I was flabbergasted! I was also a little nervous because I don't like surprises, and I especially don't like sentimentality. If only I had known how perfectly Aaron would capture my philosophy in his lovely song…

My roommate Debbie and I spent hours putting together two ambitious display boards. We covered the white board with pictures of my life: my parents, my friends, parties, school, work, and travel. The black board also had some photos, but it was more of a resume, with a timeline of my life, a few short pieces I was proud of, and lists of places I had spoken and books I had written. I felt like I was on "This Is Your Life," and it was a good feeling. I have trouble giving myself credit for the things I accomplish (they seem so small to me). This project helped with that just a little bit.

I felt strongly that I had something to say to all my guests, and I wanted it to be something that could be shared and enjoyed after the party was over. I designed a program, and inside the front cover, I wrote:

Dear Friends,

Thank you for sharing this special day with me! I want to spend an hour visiting with each one of you; but with so many people here today, chances are that I will get to speak with you only briefly. Hence, this note. For me, there are layers of significance about turning "Four-0" that I would like to share with you.

I was born in the 1960s with a disability that no one really understood. The Jerry Lewis Telethon and the death of so many of *my classmates, combined with my repeated bouts of pneumonia, gave me a subtle but powerful message that I would not live very long. My parents never bought into it, though. They made plans for my college education, and wanted me to plan, too.*

So I did, with a vengeance! Some might view their own mortality as a reason for fear or sadness. To me, it meant that if I was going to make a difference in the world, I had better start soon and not let up. As time has gone by, and more of my friends have passed away, my appreciation for this gift called LIFE has only grown. My body has weakened, but with the support of my personal assistants and friends, and with amazing advances in technology, I am healthier and happier than ever before. I have been pondering the possibility of turning 50... 60... 70? Who knows? All bets are off.

Let us enjoy every day, and never take it for granted. Thank you for coming… Thank you for caring… Thank you for being a part of my life!

Before I was ready, the day arrived: June 2, 2002. Of course I was obsessing about everything I had hoped to do that didn't get done… but we had people, delicious food, beautiful flowers, balloons and banners, lots of cameras and video equipment, and our wonderful singers! It was a great day. For me, it was a blur of conversation and laughter, people hugging me and each other, food being enjoyed, and everyone listening in rapt attention to the music…

I had planned out the six songs that Janice and Aaron were going to perform. Some were funny ("How do I know my youth is all spent? My get-up-and-go has got up and went"), while others were more serious ("Wind Beneath My Wings"). A few days before the party, I was alerted that a surprise was in the works, but that I would like it. Near the end of the program, Aaron started singing "You've Got a Friend." That wasn't on my list, but it is a song I like so it was fine with me. Pat and Dvora, who love to dance, began to move around the table where I was sitting. My roommate, my brother and cousin and their spouses were at the same table with me. Pat motioned others to join in the dance, and soon there was a circle of people surrounding our table, holding hands, smiling, and looking at me with love and commitment. It felt like a group hug with 30 people! It was a truly wonderful moment. The dance included some members of my circle of support, but also my former roommate Mattie, several personal assistants, and some people I had only known professionally. It was a beautiful cross-section of the important people in my life.

When my circle of support started in 1987, one of the first things I was struck by was how well all my friends got along once they all had the opportunity to meet one another. I have always had many friends, and would speak of them to one another, but when we all came together with a united goal, the thing quickly became bigger than any one of us. This party was the same way. My case workers met my teachers, who met my coworkers, who met my relatives, who met my friends, and so on.

Even when the party was over, it continued for weeks. Before I had even gotten very far in writing my thank-you notes, *people were sending me emails and notes about what a wonderful, powerful experience they had had at my party.* Here is one of the sweetest:

> *Hi Cathy,*
>
> *We just got home from a weekend trip to Canada - our niece got married on Friday! It was a beautiful ceremony, and it was so moving to see the expressions on the faces of our niece and her new husband as they exchanged vows. Both were radiant! As I sat there watching this incredible moment, I found myself thinking of your party, and of the expression I had witnessed on all our faces as your friends held hands and danced around you, singing a reminder of your importance in all our lives. It was another moment I wouldn't have missed for all the world. It was, for me, like that moment at Caitlin's wedding, a powerful reminder of the depth and the meaning and the value of true, heart-to-heart connection. In that kind of connection, and in such a moment, as much is given as is received, and the whole world literally becomes a better place. Such love cannot confine itself to one heart, or even two. It radiates and somehow alters the balance of the universe, I am convinced. I felt honored and blessed to be part of your celebration, as I do to be part of your life. What you have accomplished - and I saw this so clearly on your face, and on the*

faces of everyone in that circle - is a way of BEING in the world and in your relationships which is transformative. It was not what you DID at the party (i.e., how the party was organized, who you spoke with, who you didn't, etc.) but simply who you ARE, that made us all glad to be there. So, in fact, I am wanting to thank you for being you, and for the opportunity to celebrate you at your wonderful party! I was touched by the day.

Julie

Three women ended up at a table together, and in the course of their discussion realized that each had lost a close family member in the last six months. They supported one another in their grief and reaffirmed the theme that life is a gift.

Two people took the letter I had written in my program and used it in a presentation. One was a high school principal who shared it with the Friday Assembly at his school. The other used it at a ceremony to award a scholarship in memory of a close relative. Someone also told me that she carries my program in her purse because she found the letter so encouraging. For weeks I would run into people at work, and they would say something like "That party was awesome. I met someone I have talked to on the phone but never seen before!"

I doubt that the ripples from this party will subside any time soon, and I feel privileged to have been part of such an amazing event.

I want to leave you with the words of the song Aaron wrote for me. Although he may not have realized it, in describing my philosophy of life, he also captured the spirit of One Candle Power.

Life is a Gift

Aaron M. Levy

Would you know what you know
Would you have learned all that you've learned
If you'd been someone else
If the tables had been turned

Would you have loved the way you've loved
Would you have brought the joy you've brought
Had you been shown a different road
Would you have taught all those you've taught, that…

Life is a gift, that you were given so you can give
You were meant for a time like this
Life is a gift to be shared with everyone
It's a gift that goes on and on and on and on and on
Your life is a gift

Would you have traveled far and wide
And known the people that you've known
People who've meant so much to who you are
People you've learned from and who you've shown, that…

Life is a gift, that you were given so you can give
You were meant for a time like this
Life is a gift to be shared with everyone
It's a gift that goes on and on and on and on and on
Your life is a gift

If the winds of change should set your ship adrift
Remember that life is a gift
If the ground beneath your feet should start to shift
Remember that life is a gift

© 2002

RESOURCES

Many people have impressed us with their work, their thoughts, or their writings about building positive communities in which all people are empowered and included. The principles for bringing peace and harmony on a large scale also work on a personal level, in living rooms, classrooms, and job sites everywhere.

On the following pages are a number of sources where you can expand your understanding of the concepts you have read about in this book. In many cases, we have ongoing and productive relationships with these organizations and individuals. Several of them were recommended by people whose opinions we value, but we have not had the opportunity to work with them directly.

Some resources defied our ability to put them into categories. Many appear in the large "General Information" section. Others which have resources in several areas may have multiple listings.

There is much more available than this list here (each web site may have 20 articles of interest, as well as additional links). However, this will give you a place to start. We hope you continue exploring the process of One Candle Power, and that you use it to make a real difference in people's lives.

GENERAL INFORMATION

Allen, Shea & Associates provides professional services in the area of planning, research, training, materials development, and evaluation within the field of human services with an emphasis on people with developmental disabilities.

> Allen, Shea & Associates
> 1780 Third Street
> Napa, CA 94559 USA
> Phone: 707-258-1326
> Fax: 707-258-8354
> Email: asa@napanet.net.
> Web site: www.allenshea.com

Circles Network is a national voluntary organization based around the key principles of Inclusion and Person Centered Planning. The organization provides unique personal support for people who are in danger of becoming socially excluded, or who are currently suffering the consequences of prior segregation and discrimination. The Circles Network facilitates inclusion in the community, primarily through the setting up of circles of support and through individual projects for specific areas of need.

> Mandy Neville
> Circles Network
> Potford's Dam Farm
> Coventry Road
> Cawston
> Rugby, Warwickshire CV23 9JP UK
> Phone: 01788 816671
> Fax: 01788 816672
> Email: mandy.neville@btopenworld.com
> Web site: www.circlesnetwork.org.uk

Communitas is one of the foundation teams under Circles of Support. George Ducharme, Pat Beeman, Pat Jackson..and more. This book is part of their learning, but only a part. They are an outstanding resource - for thinking, presentations, problem solving.

> Communitas
> P.O. Box 358

Manchester, CT. 06045-0358
tel: 860-645-6976
E-mail: George.Ducharme@dartmouth.edu

CommunityWorks is a resource for independent facilitators working for communities in which every individual is cherished... David and Faye Wetherow have long been involved in innovative service development, training and facilitation in the field of community living. As independent facilitators and teachers, they conduct planning, training and design sessions for individuals and families, government and community agencies, schools, parent associations and self-advocacy groups throughout the United States and Canada. They share their lives with an adopted daughter who has complex mobility and communication challenges.

CommunityWorks
911 Terrien Way
Parksville, BC V9P1T2 CANADA
Phone: 250-248-2531
Fax: 250-248-2685
Cell: 250-54-5113
Web site: www.community-works.net

Inclusion Distribution UK: Kevin Reeves has created a wonderful small distribution organization focused on Inclusion. He carries a range of books and videos - an excellent resource center in UK.

Inclusion Distribution UK
29 Heron Drive
Poynton, Stockport, SK12 1QR England
Phone: 0162 585-9146
Email: kreeves@inclusiononline.co.uk
Fax 01625 269243
Web: www.inclusiononline.co.uk

Inclusive Solutions: Colin Newton and Derek Wilson *are experienced educational psychologists who specialise in mainstream inclusion and co-founders of Inclusive Solutions. Together they have a combined experience of over 40 years experience as educational psychologists working across the UK. Most recently* as Principal and Senior strategic Educational Psychologists in Nottingham City LEA, they bring a wealth of practical, applied solutions and processes from their work with children and young people with exceptional needs aged between 0-19. Colin and Derek collaborated in the writing of **Circles of Friends** – a book on implementing Circles of Friends – particularly in schools.

Inclusive Solutions
49 Northcliffe Avenue,
Nottingham, NG3 6DA England
Phone: 0115 9556045 or 0115 9605071
Email: inclusive.solutions@ntlworld.com
Web: inclusive-solutions.com

The Institute for Community Inclusion (ICI) *develops resources and supports for people with disabilities and their families, fostering interdependence, productivity, and inclusion in school and community settings. ICI provides training and consultation, services, and research and dissemination in areas such as*

- employing people with disabilities in community settings
- supporting children and young adults with special health care needs
- accessing general education, and transition from school to adult life
- expanding local recreation & school activities to include people with disabilities
- promoting technology that aids participation in school/community/work
- building organizations' ability to serve culturally diverse people with disabilities
- examining the impact of national and state policies on people with disabilities and their families

John Butterworth
Institute for Community Inclusion/UCE
University of Massachusetts Boston
GCOE, 100 Morrissey Boulevard
Boston, Massachusetts 02125-3393 USA
Phone: 617-287-7645
Fax: 617-287-7664
TTY: 617-287-7597
Email: john.butterworth@umb.edu
Web site: www.communityinclusion.org

Norman Kunc and Emma Van der Klift have spent the last 20 years working to ensure that people with disabilities are able to take their rightful place in schools, workplaces, and communities. Since 1990, they have provided in-service and training in the areas of inclusive education, employment equity, conflict resolution, and other disability rights issues. They travel extensively working with school districts, human service agencies, employers and advocacy groups. Resources include "A Credo of Support," which is available as a 5-minute video or as a poster.

> Axis Consultation & Training Ltd.
> 340 Machleary Street
> Nanaimo, British Columbia
> Canada V9R 2G9
> Phone: 250-754-9939
> Fax: 250-754-9930
> Email: normemma@normemma.com
> Web site: www.normemma.com/

The Marsha Forest Centre (formerly The Centre for Integrated Education and Community), together with Inclusion Press International and Inclusion Network, focus on the development of future leadership for inclusion through the creation of focused programs, materials and research that will create a world where Everyone Belongs.

> Inclusion Press/Inclusion Network/Jack Pearpoint
> 24 Thome Crescent
> Toronto, Ontario M6H 2S5 CANADA
> Phone: 416-658-5363
> Fax: 416-658-5067
> Email: info@inclusion.com
> Web site: www.inclusion.com

Responsive Systems Associates: John O'Brien & Connie Lyle O'Brien
Systems Change, training, systems evaluation, consultations, innovations. Responsive Systems Associates' motto is "No Pit Too Deep". John and Connie have plumbed the depths in nearly every corner of the world, and have yet to find a problem to which they could not offer some constructive advice. John and Connie are leading thinkers, writers, producers, developers and creators in the field. See Inclusion Press and Human Policy Press for many of the books by John and Connie.

Responsive Systems Associates
John O'Brien & Connie Lyle O'Brien
58 Willowwick Drive
Lithonia, GA 30038-1722 USA
Tel: (770) 987-9785
E-mail: rsa770@earthlink.net
Inclusion Press: www.inclusion.com
Human Policy Press: www.soeweb.syr.edu/thechp/
HumanPolicyPress/

Judith Snow: Leader, thinker, writer, speaker, teacher. Judith's life and career are an inspiration. She is a tremendous resource that must not be missed. Judith's book, "**What's Really Worth Doing, And How To Do It**" is available from Inclusion Press - in combination with "Front Behind the Piano: - Judith's story as told by Jack Pearpoint.

Judith Snow
108 Hallam St.
Toronto, ON M6H 1W8
Tel: 416-538-9344
E-mail: judiths@ica.net

Book: Disability is Natural, by Kathie Snow. Like gender and ethnicity, disability is simply one of many natural characteristics of being human. There have always been people with disabilities in the world, and there always will be. The greatest obstacles people with disabilities face are old attitudes that create social and environmental barriers. These barriers keep many children and adults with disabilities socially isolated, physically segregated, and excluded from the mainstream of American society. What will it take to ensure people with disabilities live real lives: being included, having friends, enjoying both the rights and responsibilities of citizenship, participating in and contributing to their communities, and, in general, living typical, ordinary lives?
A Gentle Rebellion Against Old Attitudes and Perceptions
A New Way of Thinking About People with Disabilities
It's time for revolutionary common sense!

Disability is Natural
BraveHeart Press
P. O. Box 7245

Woodland Park, CO 80863 USA
Phone: 866-948-2222 (toll-free)
Phone: 719-687-0735 (local, long-distance)
Fax: 719-687-8114
Web site: www.disabilityisnatural.com

Book: Expect the Unexpected: My Dreams and How I Got There. In this autobiography, Larry Espling examines the paths his family took when he was young to enable him, his doctors and his teachers to see beyond his cerebral palsy. He explores the difference community participation, as opposed to institutionalization, makes in the life of someone with a disability. From:

Training Resource Network, Inc.
P.O. Box 439
St. Augustine, FL 32085-0439 USA
Phone: 904-823-9800 (customer service, long-distance)
Phone: 800-210-7010 (orders only, toll-free)
Fax: 904-823-3554 (fax)
Email: customerservice@trninc.com
Web site: www.trninc.com

Song: Hunter, Tom, **Connections,** a music cassette/CD about building inclusive communities, nourishing the energy to advocate for people and work for change, celebrating the gifts and strengths in each of us, and living with great expectations that we can make good things happen. Available from :

The Song Growing Co.
1225 E. Sunset Drive, #518
Bellingham, WA 98226 USA
Phone: 206-738-0340
Email: songgrow@tomhunter.com
Web site: http://www.tomhunter.com/

Book: Pearpoint, Jack, **From Behind the Piano: Building Judith Snow's Unique Circle of Friends**; afterword: John O'Brien The story of Judith Snow and her Joshua Committee. Love, determination and hard work conquer challenges. An inspiration for anyone struggling to make a difference. Now published together with Judith Snow's book: **What's Really Worth Doing, And How to Do it.** Available from:

Inclusion Press International
24 Thome Crescent
Toronto, Ontario, Canada M6H 2S5
Phone: 416-658-5363
Fax: 416-658-5067
Email: info@inclusion.com
Web site: www.inclusion.com

Book: Schaefer, Nicola, **YES! She Knows She's Here** (the update to *Does She Know She's There?*). Nicola Schaefer's first book regaled us with the struggles of Catherine (her daughter) enroute to making a life. Now, a decade after Catherine moved into her own home in Winnipeg, that story is told as only Nicola can. A 'must read' for every family even thinking about dealing with children approaching adulthood. A powerful vision of hope, laced with reality and a liberal dash of fun. Available from:

Inclusion Press International
24 Thome Crescent
Toronto, Ontario, Canada M6H 2S5
Phone: 416-658-5363
Fax: 416-658-5067
Email: info@inclusion.com
Web site: www.inclusion.com

Book: Schwartz David B., John McKnight and Michael Kendrick, **A Story That I Heard**: A Compendium of Stories, Essays, and Poetry About People with Disabilities and American Life, 1988. 85 pages. Free of charge. Available from:

Pennsylvania Developmental Disabilities Planning Council
569 Forum Building
Harrisburg, PA 17120-0025 USA
Phone: 717-787-6057
Email: info@paddc.org
Web site: www.paddc.org

LEADERSHIP

Heider, John, **The Tao of Leadership**, Humanics Limited, Atlanta, Georgia, 1985.

Jamison, Kaleel,_**The Nibble Theory and the Kernel of Power: A Book About Leadership, Self-Empowerment and Personal Growth**, Paulist Press, New York, 1984.

Nolan, Christopher, **Under the Eye of the Clock**, Dell Publishing, New York, 1987.

O'Brien, John, **Hospitality In Depth: AAMR 10/88**, Videotape of Hospitality Conference. Available from Communitas, 730 Main Street, Manchester, CT 06040 USA.

Parnes, Sidney, **Visionizing**, D.O.K. Publishers, East Aurora, New York, 1988.

Peck, Scott M. M.D., **The Different Drum: Community Making & Peace**, Simon & Schuster, New York, 1987.

Schumacher, E.F., **Small is Beautiful (Economics as if People Mattered)**, Harper & Row Publishers, 1973.

Von Oech, Roger, **A Whack on the Side of the Head (How to Unlock Your Mind for Innovation)**, Warner Books, Inc., 1983.

FINDING CAPACITIES

Bolles, Richard, **What Color is Your Parachute?** Berkeley: Ten Speed Press, 2002.

McKnight, John, **Capacity Inventory**, The Future of Low-Income Neighborhoods and the People Who Reside There: A Capacity-Oriented Strategy for Neighborhood Development, Center for Urban Affairs and Policy Research, Northwestern University, 1988.

Mount, Beth, **Personal Futures Planning: Finding Directions for Change**, Available from Graphic Futures, Inc., 1987.

O'Connell, Mary, **The Gift of Hospitality: Opening the Doors of Community Life to People with Disabilities**, Center for Urban Affairs and Policy Research, Northwestern University and Department of Rehabilitation Services, State of Illinois, February, 1988.

Rodale Institute, Community Regeneration, **Yes I Can, A Practical Guide to Discovering How Great You Really Are,** Rodale Institute, 222 Main St., Emmaus, PA, 1988.

Siegel, Bernie, **Peace, Love and Healing**, Harper & Row Publishers, New York, 1989.

PLANNING A FUTURE: METHODS AND EXAMPLES

Circles Network is a national voluntary organization based around the key principles of Inclusion and Person Centered Planning.
See Listing under GENERAL INFORMATION

Essential Lifestyle Planning is an excellent planning tool. "As we look at supporting people in their communities, we need to remember that much of the richness of "community" comes form the relationships that we have and the rituals that celebrate and build those relationships. Despite its central function, the role of ritual is rarely discussed… For people who need substantial assistance to get through life, developing positive rituals must be a priority… Once established, however, [these rituals] should change at a pace dictated by the individual, not by the rate at which new staff arrive. The rituals must be rooted in who each individual is as well as each person's current circumstances" (from "Positive Rituals and Quality of Life" by Michael W. Smull, 1993) For information about Essential Lifestyle Planning (ELP), contact

Support Development Associates
3245 Harness Creek Road
Annapolis, MD 21403 USA
Phone: 410-626-2707
Fax: 410-626-2708
Email: mwsmull@cs.com
Web site: www.allenshea.com/friends.html

The Institute for Community Inclusion (ICI) offers a wide selection of materials:
- Building a Future: Working with the Post-High School Expectations of Students and Parents (article)
- Moving On: Planning for the Future (video)
- Building Authentic Visions: How to Support the Focus Person in Person Centered Plannning (article)
- The Most Important Member: Facilitating the Focus Person's Participation in Person Centered Planning (article)
See Listing under GENERAL INFORMATION

Inclusion Network: A new 'wing' of Inclusion Press and the Marsha Forest Centre focuses on training and workshops internationally. *Design for Change, Tools for Change, and a variety of workshops evolving from the "Creative Facilitator courses are listed on our web site: www.inclusion.com. The Network is creating teams, but most courses are presently with John O'Brien, Jack Pearpoint and their associates. Learn MAPS, PATH and other tools from the originators of the tools.*

> *For information, see The Inclusion Network:* <u>www.inclusion.com/</u>

Kathy Lee *has much experience with circles of support, person-centered planning, and related methods. She has spent many years walking with people and helping them to create new opportunities in their lives.*

> Kathy Lee
> 772 Gasteiger Road
> Meadville, PA 16335 USA
> Phone: 814-337-8146 (work)
> Email: <u>klee@toolcity.net</u>

MAPS - Making Action Plans – *is a planning process for people and organizations that begins with a story - the history. Maps has a series of questions that ask a person/organization to tell us some of the milestones on their journey, so we can get to know them, dream with them, and begin to build a plan to move in the direction of their dreams. For information, see The Marsha Forest Centre listing.*

> **The Marsha Forest Centre listing** *under General Information.*
> For information about MAPS: <u>www.inclusion.com/PI-MAPS.html</u>
> For information about PATH: <u>www.inclusion.com/PI-PATH.html</u>

The Minnesota Governor's Council on Developmental Disabilities *offers a number of resources, including:*

- **It's My Choice,** *a new 84-page workbook that will help you change the way you think about your life and the options that are available to you.*
- **Friends, A Manual for Connecting Persons with Disabilities and Community Members** *– A guide for supporting people with developmental disabilities to establish relationships with people without disabilities. Based on the premise that relationships are probably the most important aspect of our lives, Friends provides concrete suggestions about relationship building – ways to help people get better connected, maximizing*

opportunities for connections to happen, and helping to broaden and deepen personal networks.

- **It's Never Too Early, It's Never Too Late, A Booklet About Personal Futures Planning** – A guidebook that introduces personal futures planning for individuals with disabilities, their families, and advocates. Futures planning is discussed as an ongoing problem solving process that focuses on the person with disabilities, his/her desires and interests, opportunities to develop personal relationships, take on positive roles in community life, increase control over his/her own life, and learn skills to achieve these goals.

> The Minnesota Governor's Council on Developmental Disabilities
> 370 Centennial Office Building
> 658 Cedar Street
> St. Paul, Minnesota 55155 USA
> Phone: 651-296-4018
> TTY: 651-296-9962
> Fax: 651-297-7200
> Toll-free number: 1-877-348-0505
> Email: admin.dd@state.mn.us
> Web site: www.mncdd.org

Beth Mount offers many wonderful resources through her organization CapacityWorks. When she was awarded the "Award for Exemplary Achievement in Print" at the November 2001 TASH conference, her work was described this way: "Through the years, Beth Mount's artwork, publications, and posters have served to inspire us all to realize that every person with a disability is a valuable and productive member of community life. The impact of Beth's 30-year body of work has been extensive and is known throughout the world. Her work has been instrumental in helping people to find meaning in supporting people with disabilities to build their lives." Books and posters to inspire person-centered work.

> Beth Mount
> Graphic Futures
> 25 West 81st Street, #16-B
> New York, NY 10024 USA
> Phone: 212-362-9492
> Fax: 212-769-2969
> Email: GraphicFutures@Compuserve.com
> www.CapacityWorks.com

PATH is a creative planning tool which starts in the future and works backwards to an outcome of first (beginning) steps that are possible and positive. It is excellent for team building. It has been used to mediate conflicts. It is loved by people who actually want to change the ways we currently work. PATH is not for the faint of heart. It is very results oriented. Relevant for all ages and all populations. Now in use by architects, small business firms, medical professionals, aboriginal communities and organizations, as well as educators and human service providers. Developed by John O'Brien, Jack Pearpoint and Marsha Forest, PATH is one of the powerful tools you need to be a good person-centered planner. See The Marsha Forest Centre, listing under General information. For information about PATH: www.inclusion.com/PI-PATH.html

BUILDING CIRCLES OF SUPPORT

All My Life's a Circle: A book from Inclusion Press introducing the basic ideas under Circles, MAPS and PATH. A good start up resource.

>   See Listing for Inclusion Press/The Marsha Forest Centre
>   under GENERAL INFORMATION

Circles Network is a national voluntary organization based around the key principles of Inclusion and Person Centered Planning.

>   See Listing under GENERAL INFORMATION

Mary Clare Carlson is an Outreach and Training Specialist for People First Wisconsin. For nearly 20 years, she has worked and trained with self-advocates, their parents, families and friends, service providers and members of the community in Wisconsin and around the country. She has received local, state, and national recognition for her work in Personal Futures Planning and Circles of Friends.

>   Mary Clare Carlson
>   People First Wisconsin
>   3195 South Superior Street
>   Milwaukee, WI 53207 USA
>   Phone: 414-483-2546 (work)
>   Email: mccarlso@execpc.com

Her book, **Stories of Circles, Circles of Stories** is published by:

>   The Wisconsin Council on Developmental Disabilities
>   722 Williamson Street
>   P.O. Box 7851
>   Madison, WI 53707 USA
>   Phone: 608-266-7826

Circles of Friends: In 1999 Colin and Derek collaborated in the writing of Circles of Friends – a book on implementing Circles of Friends – particularly in schools in UK. This book describes a simple but powerful approach to the intentional building of relationships in mainstream school settings around pupils and students at risk of exclusion or segregation because of their disability or difference. Provides a step-by-step approach to setting up peer supports and harnessing the problem solving skills of the most natural resource available to schools - other children. PRICE £14.95. Available from Amazon.co.uk.

See Listing for Inclusive Solutions under GENERAL INFORMATION

Circles Network is a national voluntary organization based around the key principles of Inclusion and Person Centered Planning.

See Listing under GENERAL INFORMATION

Kathy Lee has much experience with circles of support.

See Listing under GENERAL INFORMATION

O'Connell, Mary, **The Gift of Hospitality: Opening the Doors of Community Life to People with Disabilities**, Center for Urban Affairs and Policy Research, Northwestern University and Department of Rehabilitation Services, State of Illinois, 1988.

Perske, Robert, **Circles of Friends**, Nashville, TN: Abingdon Press, 1988.

Wolfensberger, Wolf, **A Guideline on Protecting the Health and Lives of Patients in Hospitals, Especially If the Patient Is a Member of a Societally Devalued Class**, 1992. Any time someone is admitted to a hospital, there is the danger that the person will be misunderstood and unintentionally injured. If the person has a disability, the danger is magnified. This small book contains much wisdom friends can use to protect someone during a hospital stay. Available from:

Amazon at www.theraed.com/store/bookssz.htm or,
Training Institute for Human Services Planning, Leadership, and Change Agentry
805 South Crouse Avenue
Syracuse, NY 13244-2280 USA
Phone: 315-443-4264

BUILDING BRIDGES TO THE COMMUNITY

All in the Family, *60 Minutes* program aired March 31, 2002. Profile of Geel, Belgium, a small town where people with psychiatric disabilities are supported informally in family homes and fully able to give their gifts to their community. A psychiatrist who studied Geel's attitude toward people with psychiatric disabilities describes it this way: "It's not just the treatment of the patients and the fact that they're integrated in the town. It is the impact on the rest of the community... [where a population treated with disdain elsewhere in the world] is accepted, tolerated, welcomed.... A population that treats the mentally ill with such acceptance, with such tolerance, is a tolerant community. It's a community defined by its inclusiveness rather than its exclusiveness. And I think that's quite beautiful." Available from

> Burrelle's Transcripts
> P.O. Box 7
> Livingston, NJ 07039-0007 USA
> Phone: 800-777-TEXT (8398)
> Email: transcripts@burrelles.com.
> Web site: www.burrelles.com/indextvr.html

Bellah, Robert N., **Habits of the Heart**, University of California Press, 1985.

Berkowitz, Bill, **Community Impact: Creating Grass-Roots Change in Hard Times,** Impact Publishers, San Luis Obispo, CA, 1984.

Berkowitz, Bill, **Community Dreams: Ideas for Enriching Neighborhood and Community Life**, Impact Publishers, San Luis Obispo, CA, 1984.

CommunityWorks - David and Faye Wetherow
          See Listing under GENERAL INFORMATION

DeTouqueville, Alexis, **Democracy in America,** Penguin/Mentor paperback.

DeVinck, Christopher, **The Power of the Powerless**, Doubleday, NY, 1988.

Downey, Michael, **A Blessed Weakness: The Spirit of Jean Vanier & L'Arche**, Harper & Row Publishers, San Francisco, 1986.

Groce, Nora, **Everybody Here Spoke Sign Language**, Harvard University Press, Cambridge, MA, 1985.

Palmer, Parker J., **The Company of Strangers**, Crossroad, New York, 1986.

Rodale Institute, Regeneration Project, **Community Options; Projects you can do to regenerate your community**, Rodale Press, 33 East Minor St., Emmaus, PA, 1987.

STARTING SMALL

Fulghum, Robert, **All I Really Need To Know I Learned in Kindergarten: Uncommon Thoughts on Common Things**, Villard Books, New York, 1988.

Hunter, Tom, **Connections**, a music cassette/CD about building inclusive communities, nourishing the energy to advocate for people and work for change, celebrating the gifts and strengths in each of us, and living with great expectations that we can make good things happen. Available from:

> The Song Growing Co.
> 1225 E. Sunset Drive, #518
> Bellingham, WA 98226 USA
> Phone: 206-738-0340
> Email: songgrow@tomhunter.com
> Web site: http://www.tomhunter.com/

CHANGING SYSTEMS

CommunityWorks - David and Faye Wetherow
See Listing under GENERAL INFORMATION

Inclusion Network: A new 'wing' of Inclusion Press and the Marsha Forest Centre focuses on training and workshops internationally. *Design for Change, Tools for Change, and a variety of workshops evolving from the "Creative Facilitator courses are listed on our web site: www.inclusion.com. The Network teams are led by John O'Brien, Jack Pearpoint and their associates. Interested in the challenges of change? Think Design for Change. For information, see The Inclusion Network:* www.inclusion.com/

Norman Kunc and Emma Van der Klift
See Listing under GENERAL INFORMATION

The National Program Office on Self-determination *provides information and networking on issues related to the self-determination movement for people with disabilities in all aspects of life. The self-determination movement was founded on four basic American principles: FREEDOM: the exercise of the same rights as all citizens. People with disabilities with assistance when necessary will establish where they want to live, with whom they want to live and how their time will be occupied... AUTHORITY: the control over whatever sums of money are needed for one's own support... This is accomplished through the development of an individual budget that "moves" with the person. SUPPORT: the organization of these resources as determined by the person with a disability. This means that individuals do not receive "supervision" and "staffing." Rather, folks with disabilities may seek companionship for support and contract for any number of discrete tasks for which they need assistance. RESPONSIBILITY: the wise use of public dollars. Dollars are now being used as an investment in a person's life and not handled as resources to purchase services or slots. Responsibility includes the ordinary obligations of American citizens and allows individuals to contribute to their communities in meaningful ways.*

The National Program Office on Self-determination
Institute on Disability
7 Leavitt Lane, Suite 101
Durham, NH 03824-3522 USA

Web site: www.self-determination.org

McKnight, John, "Do No Harm: A Policymaker's Guide to Evaluating Human Services and Their Alternatives", Center for Urban Research and Policy Affairs, Northwestern University, Evanston, Illinois, 1988.

McKnight, John, Professionalized Service and Disabling Help, Center for Urban Affairs and Policy Research, Northwestern University, Evanston, Illinois.

McKnight, John, John Deere and Bereavement Counselor, Bulletin of Science Technology and Society, Volume 4, NY: Pergamon Press, 1984.

McKnight, John, Why Servanthood is Bad, The Other Side 25, 1, Jan/Feb 1989.

Responsive Systems Associates: John O'Brien & Connie Lyle O'Brien
Systems Change, training, systems evaluation, consultations, innovations. Responsive Systems Associates' motto is "No Pit Too Deep". John and Connie have plumbed the depths in nearly every corner of the world, and have yet to find a problem to which they could not offer some constructive advice. John and Connie are leading thinkers, writers, producers, developers and creators in the field. See Inclusion Press and Human Policy Press for many of the books by John and Connie.

Responsive Systems Associates
John O'Brien & Connie Lyle O'Brien
58 Willowwick Drive
Lithonia, GA 30038-1722 USA
Tel: (770) 987-9785
E-mail: rsa770@earthlink.net
Inclusion Press: www.inclusion.com
Human Policy Press: www.soeweb.syr.edu/thechp/HumanPolicyPress/

GLOSSARY

Associations – Every community is filled with people interested in art, music, sports, education, politics, and dozens of other issues and activities. Formal and informal associations are often great places to start connecting people to community. Having something in common is often the first step toward building a friendship.

Bridge-builder – Someone who uses natural and developed connections to introduce people with disabilities (or others) into associations and neighborhood groups.

Building bridges to community – The process of introducing an isolated or stigmatized person into community life. Understanding what the person needs and how his or her unique gifts may benefit others is essential in creating new relationships based on mutual support, dignity, and trust.

Capacities – People's positive characteristics, abilities, talents, and resources. The ability to look at the glass as half full instead of half empty opens up many possibilities for people, whether they have disabilities or not. See also **gifts**.

Circle facilitator – Someone who pulls together a circle of support and coordinates its activities. The facilitator may be the focus person of the circle, a friend or family member of the focus person, or someone more objective brought in from outside. Responsibilities include keeping a record of the discussion, summarizing the ideas generated, and helping people make commitments to action.

Circle member – Someone who is part of a circle of support. The members of a circle of support are usually friends, family members, co-workers, neighbors, congregation members, and sometimes service providers. The majority of people in a circle of support are not paid to be there.

Circle of support (sometimes called a circle of friends) – A group of people who agree to meet on a regular basis to assist the focus person to accomplish personal visions or goals.

Dream – A person's idea about what he or she would like life to be like in the future. Far from being a "pipe dream," a set of deeply-cherished notions can (and often does) change reality. See also **vision** and **goal**.

Facilitator – Literally, the word "facilitate" means "to make easier." For our purposes, a facilitator is someone who takes what is already there – relationships, people's gifts, people's concern for one another, policies that are being changed – and brings things together in a way that helps someone become safer, happier, more independent, and/or more connected to others. See also **circle facilitator**.

Focus person – The person at the center of a circle of support. All ideas and activities of the circle are "focused" around the desires and needs of this person (although other people in the circle may also receive support when they need it).

Gifts – The unique abilities that each person brings to the world. A person may have active gifts and talents, such as being friendly, having a good singing voice, or having a knack for gardening. He or she may have less obvious gifts, such as an ability to bring people together around a common goal, or a wonderful smile and contagious laugh. See also **capacities**.

Goal – Any personal objective worth working toward. Goals may be large, such as moving to a different place, taking a new job, or getting married; or they may be modest, such as learning about local parks or getting a cat. See also **dream** and **vision**.

Person-centered planning – A tool to help people or families think about what they want their lives to be like in the future. Traditional planning models have looked primarily at what services are available, and tried to fit the individual into available slots. By contrast, the "person-centered" approach emphasizes the needs, dreams, and capacities of the person or family. Their input is essential, and guides which actions are pursued and what services are created. There are many types of person-centered planning; these include Personal Futures Planning, MAPS, PATH, and Essential Lifestyle Planning. To obtain how-to information for these and other methods, please see the Resource section.

Person-centered team – When the majority of people in a circle of support are paid human service workers, the characteristics of this group are different from those of a community-based circle of support. Both person-centered teams and circles of support work toward a positive future for the focus person.

Trust networks – Established relationships which can be drawn upon to introduce a new person into the community. For example, if a bridge-builder already knows several people who are involved in the town historical society, that group will be more open to welcoming someone who is associated with the bridge-builder.

Vision – A view of what someone hopes the future will look like, which may include where a person wants to live, recreational and social opportunities, employment, and support system. It is a good idea to be as clear about the vision as possible, often through writing it down or drawing pictures. See also **dream** and **goal**.

Walking with – When we "work with" someone, there is the necessity of professional distance. When we "walk with" someone, we share in their journey with all of its nuances: joy, pain, frustration, waiting... The bumps in their road become our obstacles as well.

Tools for Change-the CD-Rom

70 Tools & strategies to assist your family, community or organization to deal with change as we create inclusive and diverse communities.

• Organizations • Communities • Families • People with Disability Labels • Health Workers • Educators/Teachers • Adult Educators • Universities • Trainers • Facilitators • Organizers • Negotiators • Presenters • Human Service Networks

Inclusion Press

produces user friendly books, videos and now CD's, to help create a world where 'everyone belongs'.

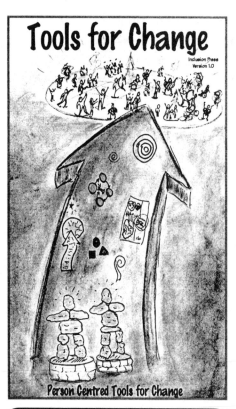

Tools for Change
Inclusion Press
Version 1.0

Person Centred Tools for Change

It's about Inclusion, Diversity & Community

* Intuitive Instructional format:
* 70 Tools for Change
* 180 overheads ready to print
* 18 articles ready to print
* 30 video clips
* 4 slide shows
* hundreds of screen pages of instructional text & diagrams

If you responsible for training, you need this!

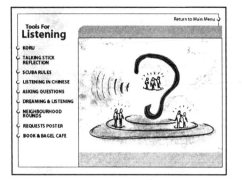

Please visit our Web site:

http://inclusion.com

for an introduction and licensing information

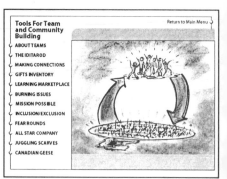

Person Centred Tools for Change

This CD is a summary of 15 years of learning, creating and collaborating between John O'Brien, Marsha Forest and Jack Pearpoint. This collection of Person Centred Strategies includes 70 tools developed by the trio to assist you to deal with change in your family

Inclusion Press

24 Thome Crescent
Toronto, ON M6H 2S5 Canada
Tel: 416-658-5363   Fax: 416-658-5067
E-mail: inclusionpress@inclusion.com

Tools for Change:
• Creativity • Planning
• Graphics • Listening
• Effective Meetings

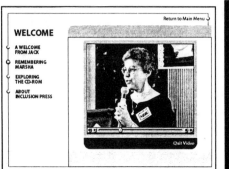

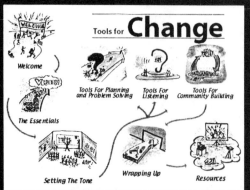

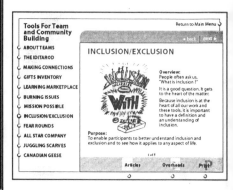

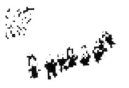

INCLUSION PRESS ORDER FORM
24 Thome Crescent, Toronto, ON Canada M6H 2S5
Tel: 416-658-5363 Fax: 416-658-5067
E-mail: inclusionpress@inclusion.com
WEBSITE: http://www.inclusion.com

Inclusion SPECIAL PACKS...

		Copies	Total
* PATH IN ACTION PACK	$150 + $15 shipping/pack	____	____
- 2 Path Training Videos [(Path in Action + Path Training) + Path Workbook]			
* All Means All PACK	$110 + $10 shipping/pack	____	____
- Video: All Means All, plus & book: All My Life's a Circle			
* Friendship PACK (1 book + Video)	$ 60 + $10 shipping/pack	____	____
- [Friendship Video + From Behind the Piano/What's Really Worth Doing]			
* Inclusion Classics Videos PACK	$ 90 + $12 shipping/pack	____	____
- Videos [With a Little Help from My Friends + Kids Belong Together]			
* Inclusion Classics Book PACK	$ 30 + $7 shipping/pack	____	____
- Books [Action for Inclusion + The Inclusion Papers]			
* Petroglyphs PACK	$ 60 + $10 shipping/pack	____	____
- Petroglyphs Book and Video on Inclusion in High Schools - from UNH			
* When Spider Webs Unite PACK	$ 80 + $10 shipping/pack	____	____
- When Spider Webs Unite - Shafik Asante - Book and Video			
** The Person-Centered Planning PACK	$ 40 + $7 shipping/pack	____	____
-2 books by O'Brien/Lyle O'Brien: Implementing Person-Centered Planning + A Little Book on Person-Centered Planning			
* The Education Book PACK	$ 40 + $7 shipping/pack	____	____
- Inclusion: Recent Research & Inclusion: How To - 2 Books - Gary Bunch			
* The Community PACK	$ 40 + $7 shipping/pack	____	____
- Members of Each Other & Celebrating the Ordinary - 2 books - John O'Brien & Connie Lyle O'Brien			

Books

		Copies	Total
** Implementing Person-Centered Planning - Voices of Experience			
Edited by John O'Brien & Connie Lyle O'Brien	$25 + $5 /1st copy shipping	____	____
** Hints for Graphic Facilitators by Jack Pearpoint	$25 + $5 /1st copy shipping	____	____
** One Candle Power by Cathy Ludlum + Communitas	$25 + $5 /1st copy shipping	____	____
A Little Book About Person Centered Planning	$20 + $5 /1st copy shipping	____	____
Forest, Lovett, Mount, Pearpoint, Smull, Snow, and Strully			
All My Life's a Circle Expanded Edition- Circles, MAPS & PATH	$20 + $5 /1st copy shipping	____	____
Path Workbook - 2nd Edition Planning Positive Possible Futures	$20 + $5 /1st copy shipping	____	____
Celebrating the Ordinary O'Brien, O'Brien & Jacob	$25 + $5 /1st copy shipping	____	____
Members of Each Other John O'Brien & Connie Lyle O'Brien	$25 + $5 /1st copy shipping	____	____
Action for Inclusion - Classic on Inclusion	$20 + $5 /1st copy shipping	____	____
The Inclusion Papers - Strategies & Stories	$20 + $5 /1st copy shipping	____	____
Lessons for Inclusion Curriculum Ideas for Inclusion in Elementary Schools	$20 + $5 /1st copy shipping	____	____
Inclusion: How To Essential Classroom Strategies - Gary Bunch	$25+ $5 /1st copy shipping	____	____
Inclusion: Recent Research G. Bunch & A. Valeo	$25 + $5 /1st copy shipping	____	____
Kids, Disabilities Regular Classrooms Gary Bunch	$20 + $5 /1st copy shipping	____	____
Reflections on Inclusive Education	$15 + $5 /1st copy shipping	____	____
Each Belongs - Hamilton Wentworth Catholic School Bd - J. Hansen	$20 + $5 /1st copy shipping	____	____
From Behind the Piano, by Jack Pearpoint AND **What's Really Worth Doing** by Judith Snow			
- Now in ONE Book *	$20 + $5 /1st copy shipping	____	____
When Spider Webs Unite Community & Inclusion- Shafik Asante	$20 + $5 /1st copy shipping	____	____
Yes! She Knows She's Here Nicola Schaefer's NEW Book	$20 + $5 /1st copy shipping	____	____
Dream Catchers & Dolphins Marsha Forest and Jack Pearpoint	$20 + $5 /1st copy shipping	____	____
It Matters - Lessons from my Son - Janice Fialka	$15 + $5 /1st copy shipping	____	____
Do You Hear What I Hear? - Janice Fialka & Karen Mikus	$15 + $5 /1st copy shipping	____	____
The Careless Society - John McKnight	$25 + $5 /1st copy shipping	____	____

Item	Price		
Who Cares - David Schwartz	$30 + $5 /1st copy shipping	____	____
The All Star Company - Team Building by Nick Marsh	$20 + $5 /1st copy shipping	____	____
Changes in Latitudes/Attitudes Role of the Inclusion Facilitator	$20 + $5 /1st copy shipping	____	____
Petroglyphs - Inclusion in High School from UNH	$20 + $5 /1st copy shipping	____	____
Treasures - from UNH	$20 + $5 /1st copy shipping	____	____
Circle of Friends by Bob & Martha Perske	$25 + $5 /1st copy shipping	____	____
Unequal Justice by Bob Perske	$25 + $5 /1st copy shipping	____	____
Perske - Pencil Portraits 1971-1990	$30 + $5 /1st copy shipping	____	____
Inclusion – Exclusion Poster (18 X 24)	$10 + $5 /1st copy shipping	____	____
Inclusion News (free with book order)		____	____
Inclusion News in Bulk (box of 100)	$50 – includes shipping in NA	____	____

Videos & CD-ROM

TOOLS FOR CHANGE - The CD-Rom for Person Centred Planning _____

Pricing is dependent on a licensing agreement. To obtain licensing information check our website, e-mail or call us.

Item	Price		
ReDiscovering MAPS Charting Your Journey -brand NEW MAPS training video	$100 + $8 shipping /1st copy	____	____
PATH IN ACTION Working with Groups -Training Video for Path with Groups	$100 + $8 shipping /1st copy	____	____
PATH TRAINING Video Intro Training Video - An Individual Path {Joe's Path}	$75 + $8 shipping /1st copy	____	____
PATH Demo Video Univ of Dayton Ohio - Video of Workshop on PATH	$55 + $8 shipping /1st copy	____	____
Celebrating Marsha (32 minutes of edited clips from Oct.7,2001)	$50 + $8 shipping /1st copy	____	____
Each Belongs (30 years of Inclusion-15 min. celebration in Hamilton)	$50 + $8 shipping /1st copy	____	____
All Means All - Inclusion Video Introduction to Circles, MAPS and PATH	$100 + $8 shipping /1st copy	____	____
When Spider Webs Unite - Video Shafik Asante in Action	$75 + $8 /1st copy shipping	____	____
EVERYONE Has a GIFT John McKnight - Building Communities of Capacity	$75 + $8 shipping /1st copy	____	____
NEW MAPS TRAINING Video Shafik's MAP - MAPS Process - Step by Step	$75 + $8 shipping /1st copy	____	____
Friendship Video Judith, Marsha & Jack on Friendship	$55 + $8 shipping /1st copy	____	____
Petroglyphs Video - the High School video - Companionto/images from the Petroglyphs Book - **Packaged with book - $60 + $8 shipping**	$55 + $8 shipping /1st copy	____	____
Dream Catchers (Dreams & Circles)	$55 + $8 shipping /1st copy	____	____
Miller's MAP - MAPS in Action	$55 + $8 shipping /1st copy	____	____
With a Little Help from My Friends The Classic on Circles & MAPS	$55 + $8 shipping /1st copy	____	____
Kids Belong Together - MAPS & Circles	$55 + $8 shipping /1st copy	____	____
Together We're Better (3 videos) Staff Development Kit	$175 + $12 shipping	____	____

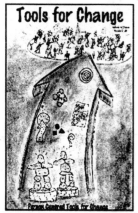

Cheques, Money Orders, Purchase Orders Please.

• Prices subject to change without notice. Shipping prices for North America only. Elsewhere by quote.

* Shipping: Books: $5 for 1st + $2/copy; Videos: $8 for 1st+ $4/copy. OR 15% of total order cost - which ever is less for customer.

Tools for Change - the CD Tools for Person Centered Planning

Plus applicable taxes (variable)

GRAND TOTAL $===========

Order NOW: TOOLS for CHANGE CD-ROM

An exciting multi-media Training Guide with resources galore for your staff. Presentation ready. A practical, usable CD-ROM featuring slide shows, graphic overheads, video clips, articles. Introduces 'tools for change' that were developed by Jack Pearpoint, Marsha Forest and John O'Brien. Essential for 'trainers' using Person Centered approaches, MAPS, PATH, Circles or just dealing with day to day change. Includes articles and overheads that can be printed.

Name: _____

Organization:_____

Address:_____

City: _____

Prov/State _____ Post Code/ZIP _____

Wk Phone _____ Cheque Enclosed _____

Hm Phone _____ Fax _____

E-Mail _____ Web Page:_____

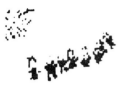

INCLUSION PRESS ORDER FORM

24 Thome Crescent, Toronto, ON Canada M6H 2S5
Tel: 416-658-5363 Fax: 416-658-5067
E-mail: inclusionpress@inclusion.com
WEBSITE: http://www.inclusion.com

Inclusion SPECIAL PACKS...

* PATH IN ACTION PACK	$150 + $15 shipping/pack	____	_____
- 2 Path Training Videos [(Path in Action + Path Training) + Path Workbook]			
* All Means All PACK	$110 + $10 shipping/pack	____	_____
- Video: All Means All, plus & book: All My Life's a Circle			
* Friendship PACK (1 book + Video)	$ 60 + $10 shipping/pack	____	_____
- [Friendship Video + From Behind the Piano/What's Really Worth Doing]			
* Inclusion Classics Videos PACK	$ 90 + $12 shipping/pack	____	_____
- Videos [With a Little Help from My Friends + Kids Belong Together]			
* Inclusion Classics Book PACK	$ 30 + $7 shipping/pack	____	_____
- Books [Action for Inclusion + The Inclusion Papers]			
* Petroglyphs PACK	$ 60 + $10 shipping/pack	____	_____
- Petroglyphs Book and Video on Inclusion in High Schools - from UNH			
* When Spider Webs Unite PACK	$ 80 + $10 shipping/pack	____	_____
- When Spider Webs Unite - Shafik Asante - Book and Video			
** The Person-Centered Planning PACK	$ 40 + $7 shipping/pack	____	_____
-2 books by O'Brien/Lyle O'Brien: Implementing Person-Centered Planning + A Little Book on Person-Centered Planning			
* The Education Book PACK	$ 40 + $7 shipping/pack	____	_____
- Inclusion: Recent Research & Inclusion: How To - 2 Books - Gary Bunch			
* The Community PACK	$ 40 + $7 shipping/pack	____	_____
- Members of Each Other & Celebrating the Ordinary - 2 books - John O'Brien & Connie Lyle O'Brien			

Books

		Copies	Total
** Implementing Person-Centered Planning - Voices of Experience			
Edited by John O'Brien & Connie Lyle O'Brien	$25 + $5 /1st copy shipping	____	_____
** Hints for Graphic Facilitators by Jack Pearpoint	$25 + $5 /1st copy shipping	____	_____
** One Candle Power by Cathy Ludlum + Communitas	$25 + $5 /1st copy shipping	____	_____
A Little Book About Person Centered Planning	$20 + $5 /1st copy shipping	____	_____
Forest, Lovett, Mount, Pearpoint, Smull, Snow, and Strully			
All My Life's a Circle Expanded Edition- Circles, MAPS & PATH	$20 + $5 /1st copy shipping	____	_____
Path Workbook - 2nd Edition Planning Positive Possible Futures	$20 + $5 /1st copy shipping	____	_____
Celebrating the Ordinary O'Brien, O'Brien & Jacob	$25 + $5 /1st copy shipping	____	_____
Members of Each Other John O'Brien & Connie Lyle O'Brien	$25 + $5 /1st copy shipping	____	_____
Action for Inclusion - Classic on Inclusion	$20 + $5 /1st copy shipping	____	_____
The Inclusion Papers - Strategies & Stories	$20 + $5 /1st copy shipping	____	_____
Lessons for Inclusion Curriculum Ideas for Inclusion in Elementary Schools	$20 + $5 /1st copy shipping	____	_____
Inclusion: How To Essential Classroom Strategies - Gary Bunch	$25+ $5 /1st copy shipping	____	_____
Inclusion: Recent Research G. Bunch & A. Valeo	$25 + $5 /1st copy shipping	____	_____
Kids, Disabilities Regular Classrooms Gary Bunch	$20 + $5 /1st copy shipping	____	_____
Reflections on Inclusive Education	$15 + $5 /1st copy shipping	____	_____
Each Belongs - Hamilton Wentworth Catholic School Bd - J. Hansen	$20 + $5 /1st copy shipping	____	_____
From Behind the Piano, by Jack Pearpoint AND **What's Really Worth Doing** by Judith Snow			
- Now in ONE Book *	$20 + $5 /1st copy shipping	____	_____
When Spider Webs Unite Community & Inclusion- Shafik Asante	$20 + $5 /1st copy shipping	____	_____
Yes! She Knows She's Here Nicola Schaefer's NEW Book	$20 + $5 /1st copy shipping	____	_____
Dream Catchers & Dolphins Marsha Forest and Jack Pearpoint	$20 + $5 /1st copy shipping	____	_____
It Matters - Lessons from my Son - Janice Fialka	$15 + $5 /1st copy shipping	____	_____
Do You Hear What I Hear? - Janice Fialka & Karen Mikus	$15 + $5 /1st copy shipping	____	_____
The Careless Society - John McKnight	$25 + $5 /1st copy shipping	____	_____

Who Cares - David Schwartz	$30 + $5 /1st copy shipping	____	____
The All Star Company - Team Building by Nick Marsh	$20 + $5 /1st copy shipping	____	____
Changes in Latitudes/Attitudes Role of the Inclusion Facilitator	$20 + $5 /1st copy shipping	____	____
Petroglyphs - Inclusion in High School from UNH	$20 + $5 /1st copy shipping	____	____
Treasures - from UNH	$20 + $5 /1st copy shipping	____	____
Circle of Friends by Bob & Martha Perske	$25 + $5 /1st copy shipping	____	____
Unequal Justice by Bob Perske	$25 + $5 /1st copy shipping	____	____
Perske - Pencil Portraits 1971-1990	$30 + $5 /1st copy shipping	____	____
Inclusion – Exclusion Poster (18 X 24)	$10 + $5 /1st copy shipping	____	____
Inclusion News (free with book order)		____	____
Inclusion News in Bulk (box of 100)	$50 – includes shipping in NA	____	____

Videos & CD-ROM

TOOLS FOR CHANGE - The CD-Rom for Person Centred Planning ____

Pricing is dependent on a licensing agreement. To obtain licensing information check our website, e-mail or call us.

ReDiscovering MAPS Charting Your Journey -brand NEW MAPS training video	$100 + $8 shipping /1st copy	____	____
PATH IN ACTION Working with Groups -Training Video for Path with Groups	$100 + $8 shipping /1st copy	____	____
PATH TRAINING Video Intro Training Video - An Individual Path {Joe's Path}	$75 + $8 shipping /1st copy	____	____
PATH Demo Video Univ of Dayton Ohio - Video of Workshop on PATH	$55 + $8 shipping /1st copy	____	____
Celebrating Marsha (32 minutes of edited clips from Oct.7,2001)	$50 + $8 shipping /1st copy	____	____
Each Belongs (30 years of Inclusion-15 min. celebration in Hamilton)	$50 + $8 shipping /1st copy	____	____
All Means All - Inclusion Video Introduction to Circles, MAPS and PATH	$100 + $8 shipping /1st copy	____	____
When Spider Webs Unite - Video Shafik Asante in Action	$75 + $8 /1st copy shipping	____	____
EVERYONE Has a GIFT John McKnight - Building Communities of Capacity	$75 + $8 shipping /1st copy	____	____
NEW MAPS TRAINING Video Shafik's MAP - MAPS Process - Step by Step	$75 + $8 shipping /1st copy	____	____
Friendship Video Judith, Marsha & Jack on Friendship	$55 + $8 shipping /1st copy	____	____
Petroglyphs Video - the High School video - Companionto/images from the Petroglyphs Book - Packaged with book - $60 + $8 shipping	$55 + $8 shipping /1st copy	____	____
Dream Catchers (Dreams & Circles)	$55 + $8 shipping /1st copy	____	____
Miller's MAP - MAPS in Action	$55 + $8 shipping /1st copy	____	____
With a Little Help from My Friends The Classic on Circles & MAPS	$55 + $8 shipping /1st copy	____	____
Kids Belong Together - MAPS & Circles	$55 + $8 shipping /1st copy	____	____
Together We're Better (3 videos) Staff Development Kit	$175 + $12 shipping	____	____

Cheques, Money Orders, Purchase Orders Please.
- Prices subject to change without notice. Shipping prices for North America only. Elsewhere by quote.

* Shipping: Books: $5 for 1st + $2/copy; Videos: $8 for 1st+ $4/copy. OR 15% of total order cost - which ever is less for customer.

Tools for Change - the CD
Tools for Person Centered Planning

Plus applicable taxes (variable)

GRAND TOTAL $===========

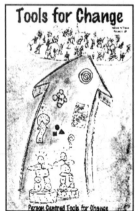

Order NOW: TOOLS for CHANGE CD-ROM
An exciting multi-media Training Guide with resources galore for your staff. Presentation ready. A practical, usable CD-ROM featuring slide shows, graphic overheads, video clips, articles. Introduces 'tools for change' that were developed by Jack Pearpoint, Marsha Forest and John O'Brien. Essential for 'trainers' using Person Centered approaches, MAPS, PATH, Circles or just dealing with day to day change. Includes articles and overheads that can be printed.

Name: _____
Organization:_____
Address:_____
City: _____
Prov/State _____ Post Code/ZIP _____
Wk Phone _____ Cheque Enclosed _____
Hm Phone _____ Fax _____
E-Mail _____ Web Page:_____